W9-BMJ-018

CREATIVE SUFFERING

Creative Suffering

PAUL TOURNIER

HARPER & ROW, PUBLISHERS, San Francisco
Cambridge, Hagerstown, New York, Philadelphia
London, Mexico City, São Paulo, Sydney

CREATIVE SUFFERING. First published in France as
Face a la souffrance. Copyright © 1981 by Editions
Labour et Fides. Translation copyright © 1982 by
Edwin Hudson. All rights reserved. Printed in the
United States of America. No part of this book may
be used or reproduced in any manner whatsoever
without written permission except in the case of
brief quotations embodied in critical articles and
reviews. For information address Harper & Row,
Publishers, Inc., 10 East 53rd Street, New York,
NY 10022. Published simultaneously in Canada by
Fitzhenry & Whiteside, Limited, Toronto.

FIRST U.S. EDITION

Library of Congress Cataloging in Publication Data

Tournier, Paul.
  CREATIVE SUFFERING.

  Translation of: Face à la souffrance.
  Bibliography: p.
  1. Suffering—Religious aspects—Christianity. I. Title.
BT732.7.T6813   1983   231'.8   82-48939
ISBN 0-06-068296-5

83 84 85 86 87 10 9 8 7 6 5 4 3 2 1

To Dr Klaus Thomas of Berlin,
and Pastor Raynald Martin of Geneva,
who pioneered the Helpline Telephone Service,
and to all their fellow-workers,
and also to Drs Pierre Rentchnick and André Haynal,
whose work inspired me to write this book.

CONTENTS

Prologue: The Enigma of the Orphan   1

1 A Link Between Deprivation and Creativity   7

2 A Blessing in Disguise?   22

3 Win or Lose?   39

4 Deprivation and Frustration   55

5 The Difficulties and Delays of Acceptance   68

6 Anger   81

7 Courage   94

8 Noise, in the Theory of Information   111

9 Routine and Creativity   125

List of Works Quoted   141

Prologue:
The Enigma of the Orphan

When I start writing a book I always picture you, my unknown reader, as you open it at this first page. This is my twentieth book: a sort of jubilee. And so you come close to me, seeking that dialogue with the author which reading a book always involves. But we are not yet quite together: you are joining me at this point in my thoughts on my subject, but for me this point is the culmination of a long process made up of many personal experiences, many surprises, and many confidences received: a long journey of which you know nothing. I too am seeking contact with you, but I know nothing about you either. Your reactions to what I write will depend on your own experiences, especially if you are in trouble or have known adversity. There is a risk that something I say will re-open the wound.

Therefore, since I cannot share your life, I must tell you something about my own, and then you can follow me along that bit of my road which has brought me now to this book. My starting-point was an article written by Dr Pierre Rentchnick of Geneva, which appeared in the periodical *Médecine et hygiène*, of which he is the editor, on 26 November 1975, under the surprising title, 'Orphans Lead the World'. When President Pompidou died, my colleague found himself wondering what might have been the political repercussions of disease in the case of other statesmen, such as for example President Roosevelt at the end of the war. So he set about reading the life-stories of the politicians who had had the greatest influence on the course of world history.

He was soon struck by the astonishing discovery that all of them had been orphans! Some had lost their fathers in infancy or in early youth, others their mothers, and some both parents, or else they had been cut off from one or the other because they had separated; or else they had been illegitimate children and had not known their fathers or anything about them. Yet others had been rejected or abandoned by their parents. Dr Rentchnick compiled a list of them. It contained almost three hundred of the greatest names in history, from Alexander the Great and Julius Caesar, through Charles V, Cardinal Richelieu, Louis XIV, Robespierre, George Washington, Napoleon, Queen Victoria, Golda Meir, Hitler, Lenin, Stalin, to Eva Perón, Fidel Castro, and Houphouet-Boigny.

These are only a few examples – obviously I cannot enumerate here the names of all those famous people, carefully classified by the author, who illustrates his article with their portraits: all of them had suffered in childhood from emotional deprivation. He informed me that the only two exceptions he had come across were Chancellor Bismarck and General De Gaulle. Even so I found Bismarck in his list of those deserted in childhood.

So there we are, giving lectures on how important it is for a child's development to have a father and a mother performing harmoniously together their respective roles towards him. And all at once we find that this is the very thing that those who have been most influential in world history have not had! From this surprising revelation my colleague deduced 'a new theory of the genesis of the will to political power': the insecurity consequent upon emotional deprivation must have aroused in these children an exceptional will to power, which drove them into a career in politics with the aim of 'transforming the world', and succeeding in so far as they were able.

Of course I was particularly interested in this article, since I was an orphan myself, my father having died when I was two months old, and my mother when I was five. I went to see my colleague to talk about it. It was soon after my wife's death, I now realize, and I felt as if I had been orphaned for the third time. Although I had always thought of myself as pacific and conciliatory, I had to admit that unconsciously I was actuated by a quite exceptional will to power. True, I had taken no part in politics, but I had a keen interest in political matters in my student days. In fact only recently I chanced to meet an old friend in a tram, and between two stops we recalled together the good old days of our youth, and as he got off he called to me from the pavement, 'You know, we were all sure you would be President of Switzerland one day!' Fortunately for me, regulations had prevented me from taking the first step and standing for the cantonal parliament, since at that time I was a hospital doctor, and as a paid servant of the State I was ineligible.

However, in taking up medicine I was entering upon a career of power just as surely as if I had been a politician. Emmanuel Mounier called it the 'fourth power'. The whole of the satisfaction we get out of it is bound up with our power against disease and death. And when we feel we are losing the battle we have chosen to engage in, our disappointment and humiliation leaves us downcast. But there is more to it than that: it gives us power over people, over our patients when they give us that unconditional confidence which is so important to us; and our power over the nurses and the others who work with us; over the whole medical team in the case of the director of a large hospital; and even over the most high-and-mighty bureaucrat, who must bow to a medical certificate. One might also mention the collusion of doctors with powerful pharmaceutical firms, which Illich denounces in his *Medical Nemesis*.

Most doctors tend not to realize the power they wield, so accustomed are they to being listened to without question; nor do they realize the harmful effect it has on their own characters. Sometimes it is the doctor's wife who notices it, without being able to say anything – her job is to see to the unlimited devotion of the whole family to the career of a father who is himself so devoted to his patients. It can happen that a patient, accustomed to the doctor's kindly and benevolent attitude, thinks he ought to tell him that the medicine he has prescribed does not suit him, and is astonished to see him fly into a violent temper. Why is it that the doctor – a man of science, after all – refuses to take into account the evidence of his own experience?

My vocation, however, is not solely a medical one, and I talked to Dr Rentchnick about my religious vocation, of which he was not unaware. He exclaimed triumphantly, 'The great religious leaders were orphans, too! Remember Moses floating in his basket on the waters of the Nile!' In *Moses and Monotheism* Freud suggests that Moses was actually the son of the tender-hearted princess who found him so opportunely among the reeds, and took him as a stranger to the palace of the Pharaoh, her father. However that may be, Moses was an abandoned child, and this may well be the explanation of his violence in killing an Egyptian. The Buddha, too, was an orphan, as was Mahomet, whose father and mother both died before he was one year old!

It is not difficult to imagine the sense of power a man may have when he feels called to speak in God's name, and when he is listened to as God's spokesman. Or even when he expounds

4

a truth as a philosopher. Dr Rentchnick had therefore included among the names of statesmen those of religious leaders and philosophers. He referred to Jean-Paul Sartre's *Words*, in which he talks about his childhood as an orphan. We are familiar with the prestige that great preachers and philosophers have always enjoyed, and we recognize that it is due not only to their inspired teaching but also to their qualities as leaders of men. Confucius lost his father at the age of one, Rousseau his mother shortly after his birth, Descartes lost his at the age of one year, and Pascal at the age of three.

Thus an unconscious will to power seems to play an important part in the lives of most eminent men. This has its good aspect, since they are able to put it at the service of God, of men, and of culture. But it does not make agreement among them easy. How can one be conciliatory and tolerant when one looks upon oneself as the custodian of an eternal truth? And so religious wars and ideological revolutions are among those that are most fiercely fought. The old formula *rabies theologica*, theological madness, expresses an age-old experience. The thirst for power is capable of driving the great ones of this world – as well as each and every one of us – to the highest but also the lowest actions.

At the time of my conversation with Dr Rentchnick I happened to be engaged in writing my book *The Violence Inside*, which I might summarize as follows: How dangerous it is for a man to be powerful, since ambition and violence increase inexorably with power! I could not omit to devote a chapter to the growing power of medicine; and of course I included all this about orphans, my colleague's article, our discussion, and my thoughts on the matter. My friend in his turn developed his ideas, and published a book based on the original article. And in his book he mentions me on the very first page, which pleases me very much! Is not this rather childish game of mutual compliments played in every university, church, and drawing-room? 'I flatter you because you flattered me, and you flatter me because I flattered you,' one might say.

I

A Link Between Deprivation and Creativity

There is, however, much more in Dr Rentchnick's book, more cautiously entitled *Do Orphans Lead the World?* For my colleague had the happy idea of asking a historian and a psychoanalyst to complement his work with essays dealing with the theme in the light of their respective disciplines. The historian was Professor Pierre de Senarclens, who wrote under the title 'Is it possible to write a psychoanalytical biography of a politician?' What interests the historian is what statesmen do, their political actions, rather than why they have entered politics, the conscious or unconscious motivations of their political choices, rather than of their choice of career. It is a most interesting question, but rather different from the one put by Dr Rentchnick. Professor de Senarclens answers it in the negative: the intimate experiences of a statesman may have motivated his desire for power, but they do not explain the political use he makes of it.

The psychoanalyst is Professor André Haynal, who entitles his essay, 'A psychoanalytical discourse on deprivation, with special reference to orphans'. I devoured this treatise with enthusiasm. It is not long, however – hardly more than sixty pages. It showed me how psychoanalysis, handled with clarity and wisdom, can help us to understand the affective mechanisms which may transfigure the life of an orphan, as I had seen and experienced for myself. I was struck also by the large number of convincing examples which the author had gleaned from history and literature. But there was something else – my second surprise, the second turning-point in the journey of my thoughts on which I have invited you to accompany me.

Dr Haynal, as you have seen from his title, introduces a new idea, that of 'deprivation', and in so doing he imparts a quite new dimension to the discussion. The orphan child is deprived of one or both of his parents. But there are many other 'deprivations' in life. To begin with, as a man whom I knew well as a student wrote to me, there are so many people who have not in fact been orphaned, whose fathers are still alive, but they have become, as had his own, to all intents and purposes non-existent so far as the child is concerned. This goes much further, however. As soon as we think of deprivation our minds are filled with an endless procession of unfortunate lives.

Naturally, I think first of all those unmarried women who have confided in me, whose daily suffering in being deprived of husband and children is made all the worse by their having to hide it. They are deprived of physical love, but even more – even if they have a lover – they lack the sharing of the whole of life, the 'togetherness' which women need more than men. And even if the unmarried woman has a child, however much she loves the child the support and authority of a father is missing. Think too of all those crossed in love, and all the abandoned husbands and wives to whom the sudden departure of their partners so often comes as a shock like a bolt from the blue. And all those childless couples, and even more, those who have lost a child – a deprivation they will always feel, even though they may no longer talk about it. And all the failures life brings, all the divorces, all the bereavements.

In addition, many married women, even those with apparently harmonious marriages, suffer a more subtle but painful deprivation – the absence of any real dialogue with their husbands, because men are so bad at expressing their feelings. I mentioned one such case in my last book, *The Gift of Feeling*. A wife may talk for hours to her husband without his uttering a word in reply. And when he does answer her it is only about objective facts or abstract ideas, not about what he is feeling himself or his personal preoccupations.

There are also many people who are deprived of the most elementary things in life – food, for example, without which they will die of starvation. For many there is a lack of financial security, or of employment, and the countless refugees who have lost their homeland. And those who have longed to take up a course of study and have been unable to do so, and who bitterly carry the deprivation of it about with them for the rest of their lives; and those who have had to renounce their chosen vocation. The sick are deprived of health, the infirm are deprived of hearing or sight, or a limb, or of mobility and the independence it confers. The old lack youth, the retired miss their work and the social relationships that went with it, and which used to play such a large part in their lives. Large numbers of those who are in work find no interest in what they do; and so many people have no real friends at all. You will remember how movingly St Augustine wrote in the *Confessions* about the death of his friend, of how joy had gone out of his life, and he felt torn asunder.

Then there is the great deprivation which Viktor Frankl denounces in our Western civilization: the fact that so many of us find no meaning in our lives, even sometimes at the height of success in a career or in society. And the lack of silence, of green fields, of sunshine, of peace, of any inner life, or simply of being accepted. All those on the fringes of

9

society, homosexuals, the victims of social or natural misfortunes, those who lack the esteem of others, those who are too shy to express themselves, and the neurotics who are deprived of the love that would cure them.

You will understand that I cannot prolong this inventory. How much suffering there is in our world! We have gone far beyond the boundaries of the problem of orphans; but the analogy is clear. 'Everybody can't be an orphan,' Poil-de-Carotte says in Jules Renard's book. But Dr Haynal puts a quotation from Saul Bellow at the head of his essay: 'Everyone is born to be an orphan.' And he writes: 'Orphans merely suffer more intensely something that is a fundamental human experience.' Namely, the experience of deprivation, or of finitude, which involves us all. It involves, in fact, all the trials of life that we have to face. And even if there are some exceptionally privileged people, they are still deprived – deprived of suffering, which is necessary in order to become really human. They could be said to be deprived of deprivation.

In any case it is rare for such people to be aware of their privileged state and to enjoy it. If we are really to appreciate good weather it has to follow on a long spell of bad weather. In the same way we are better able to appreciate the good times when they come after the bad ones. Those who are privileged tend to worry much more about the things they still have not got; or even, ridiculously enough, about what they may possibly be without. Such, as we all know, is the insatiable nature of desire.

Perhaps, instead of making a higgledy-piggledy catalogue of our deprivations, it would be more appropriate to distinguish those which concern our vital needs, both material and spiritual, from the often futile desires that endlessly spring into being in our hearts. René Girard stresses the common phenomenon which he calls mimetic desire: it only needs someone else to have an advantage or a possession which we have not got, for us to covet it and to realize our lack of it. It is all very well for the moralists to tell us to be good and to assure us that happiness comes from being content with one's lot. It is easily said when one lacks nothing, which is usually the case with them. They denounce in vain the foolishness of men whose inexhaustible ambition aggravates their suffering.

I am not so severe as they are, because I think I can see in this trait a fundamental characteristic of life, which not one of us can escape so long as we live. I often think of this when I observe the exuberance of nature, when I trim the shrubs planted round my villa which grow so abundantly and so quickly. The mayor of our commune is a colleague of mine, Dr Dottrens. He was once called upon to preach in the Cathedral. He concluded his sermon with a very characteristic anecdote about the sense of wonder which the doctor always has when he observes the power of life. In the middle of the town, on a road pounded by the incessant tramp of passers-by, he had seen a tiny plant which had managed to push up the hard crust of asphalt, to crack it, and to thrust its thin shoot through the fissure to display two tender leaves triumphantly to the sun.

So long as there is life, there is desire, the desire to grow. Even the ascetic draws from this life-force the strength to remain faithful to his vows; and he denies himself in order to have the benefit of his asceticism. It is fortunate for us that this is so, for is it not on this power of nature that medicine has basically relied ever since Hippocrates? The disease – a kind of deprivation – is the obstacle, and the doctor is constantly on the lookout, waiting for life to strike back. This is even more true of us believers who know that life is the breath of God who is fighting at our side.

So our discussion has been widened through the introduction of the more general notion of deprivation. An analogy comes to mind: in the cinema, the camera shows us a close-up of a character, filling the whole screen. Suddenly, using its zoom lens, it enlarges the field of vision to the other extreme, so that the character becomes a tiny figure lost in a huge crowd. With Dr Rentchnick we have fixed our attention on the particular problem of the orphan, but with Dr Haynal we realize that that is simply a special case of the countless sufferings of life with which the doctor is confronted every day. Nevertheless the case of the orphan is particularly striking, and lends itself to study, since one either is an orphan or one is not, so that it is possible to draw up statistics. That is not possible with the other multifarious frustrations of life. It would be useless to try to establish a sort of personal coefficient of happiness or un-happiness for human beings.

But it is also the import of our argument which Dr Haynal has changed: Dr Rentchnick referred to the will to power in the case of the great orphans who had left their mark on history. Dr Haynal speaks of creativity, which is quite different. You can imagine the satisfaction with which I read that: I should rather be thought to possess a little creativity than a great will to power!

When you think about it you realize that even for a statesman the will to power is not enough. It can make a tyrant of him, a dictator who seizes power and keeps his hold on it by force. The only true political leader is one who is able to present to the masses an attractive ideal which they spontaneously accept. He is therefore a creator, even if his programme proves to be harmful. 'A politician endowed with creativity,' writes Dr Haynal, 'becomes a leader.' The author does not deny the role of the will to power, but he considers it to be an auxiliary one. Life is change, he says, and men fear change. The leader is the one who helps them to adapt to it: 'it is always a matter of doing something new'. Even in science, the genius is the man who discovers new concepts, and this is chiefly a function of creative intuition.

Not surprisingly, in the examples of creativity which he gives, the author accords much more space than does Dr Rentchnick to artists and writers. 'Several psychoanalysts, of whom I am one,' he writes, 'are convinced that there is a relationship between the processes of bereavement, loss, deprivation, and creativity. One cannot but be impressed by the high proportion of orphans one finds among creative artists.' Leonardo da Vinci was an illegitimate child, and J. S. Bach was an orphan. Among writers we have Molière, Racine, Stendhal, Baudelaire, Camus, Georges Sand, Kipling, Edgar Allen Poe, Dante, Alexandre Dumas, Tolstoy, Voltaire, Byron, Dostoievsky, and Balzac, to say nothing of Jean-Jacques Rousseau and Jean-Paul Sartre, whom I have already mentioned.

Recently I lectured on this theme in a hospital in South Africa. A young woman was acting as my interpreter, a courageous woman who had had to struggle against the consequences of polio in infancy. She was a teacher of French. Afterwards, in the car, she told me that while she was translating my speech she was thinking about her favourite French authors, and realizing that in fact they had all suffered from some handicap in childhood.

Here, however, the statistics are less conclusive. Whereas Dr Rentchnick found that almost all great statesmen were orphans, Dr Porret gives a list of eighteen famous authors who had both father and mother up to the age of twenty, including Flaubert, Chateaubriand, Lamartine, and Verlaine. Whence comes this difference? Very likely from the fact that the will to power, as Rentchnick said, plays its part in the choice of a political career. Lamartine was tempted by it, but was less successful as a politician than as a poet. There are also many doctors who have been statesmen.

Haynal also wonders why 'a creative personality chooses political action rather than expressing his aspirations in music, in the novel, or in lyric poetry'. The quality of being a good mixer, an extrovert temperament, he adds, may in part explain a preference for the 'transfer to action' of political life, over the 'meditation' of an artistic or a scientific career. There is, of course, an allusion here to the will to power. There is a great contrast between the decisiveness of the statesman and the interminable hesitations of the artist. For the latter, the 'transfer to action' is the taking up of the pen, the brush, or the chisel, and I know myself how long I can vacillate before doing so.

Statistics, therefore, seem to show that a connection between being an orphan and the choice of career is less common among artists and scientists than among political and religious leaders. But how are we to know what other deprivations have contributed in the case of the former to the awakening of their creativity? So I am not going to say anything more about statistics. I am too much of a doctor for that. What fascinates me is not so much suffering in general, but the quite particular personal suffering of the patient who is there telling me about it. I am more interested in the person than in mankind in general, or rather it is the person who reveals to me the reality of mankind better than all your sociological statistics.

The more so as a statistician would have many other questions to ask. I remember having read somewhere that in the eighteenth century the average length of time that a married couple lived together was twenty years. That means that about half their children lost at least one parent in childhood or early youth.

I began with statistics because that is what first alerted me to the problem. In fact the question that has thus been raised is that of the supposed benefit of suffering. It is a question that brings a host of memories into my mind. I think of all those who have confided in me, whose development I have followed during a particularly painful period of their lives, in sickness, bereavement, conflicts, and failures, and of how we have always found a common bond as we carried the burden together. I remember too how I have seen them change through suffering, and how that has impressed me and changed me as well. It is true that the changes were not usually the ones that either they or I expected; but I think I can say that most of them gained by their experience, as well as suffering from it.

In the street one day I meet a former patient, whose serious illness caused me a lot of worry at the time. He is obviously very pleased to meet me again, and remarks in a jocular tone that is not meant to hide his seriousness, 'Oh, doctor, you know I have very happy memories of that time. It was tough, all right, but looking back, it seems to me that it was one of the most fruitful periods of my life. I learnt more in those few months of illness than in twenty years of good health!'

It is not hard to find further examples. I open the autobiography of Edmond Kaiser, the founder of Terre des Hommes. On the first page he writes of the death of his father in the 1914 war, when he was still quite young. Further on he tells of the accidental death of his son with such feeling that one realizes that the pain is still acute, and that he is still tormented by remorse because he had done nothing to forestall that misfortune. But it is clear that that was what led him to create the organization which has saved thousands of children from death.

I read the book in which Anwar El Sadat recounts his life. The most impressive chapter is the account of the year he spent in prison when he was fighting the British for the independence of his country. He reveals his inner struggle in that solitude to discover his own identity and the rules of conduct that had to guide and inspire him in the courageous acts that were to come.

That reminds me of Dr Roberto Assagioli of Florence, who also spent a year in prison under Mussolini, because he was of Jewish race, though a Catholic. During one of our sessions on the medicine of the person he amused us by remarking that it was the best year of his life, because there was no telephone in his prison cell. But behind the jocular remark one could sense that it was during that year that he evolved the method of psychosynthesis for which he is famous both in the United States and in Europe.

Historical examples are not hard to find. Mention of creativity turns one's thoughts to the Renaissance. The very name, and the thought of all the treasures of literature and art that it conjures up, tend to make us picture the Renaissance as a kind of golden age in which writers and artists, excited by the discovery of the masterpieces of antiquity, could devote themselves peacefully to their arts. However, a specialist in the period, Jean Delumeau of the Collège de France, describes it as one of the most sinister and terrifying eras in the whole of history. There was the constant menace of the Turks, epidemic plagues, roving bands of armed men, witch-hunts, and cruel religious wars.

The church, up to then one of the pillars of society, was torn asunder by the schism of the Reformation. Both Catholics and Protestants, he says, expected the imminent and apocalyptic end of the world. Panic reigned throughout Europe, and it was in this climate of despair that the foundations of modern thought were laid, and the scientific method, which has been so productive, was evolved, while artists surpassed themselves.

Similarly the greatest flowering of Greek thought, the age of Socrates, Plato, and Aristotle, did not coincide with the period of Athens' greatest power, but came after its disastrous defeat in the Peloponnesian War which sealed its fate. In Jerusalem, it was under the imminent threat of the foreign invasion that was to destroy it that Jeremiah arose. It was among the despairing exiles in Mesopotamia that the prophetic song of the second Isaiah was heard, and Ezekiel's assertion that the dry bones would live again. Jesus himself was born under the harshest of political regimes, that of brutal foreign occupation. We know what that means, and I understand what André Chouraqui has to say about the responsibility of the Romans for Christ's crucifixion – a responsibility which obviously no narrator of the time dared to denounce.

We Swiss celebrate the heroic times when our country was founded 'in the name of almighty God', the period of the wars of independence, and we know well what sufferings and what sacrifices it had to endure in order to win that independence and then to establish it in the middle of a continent torn by the conflicts of the great powers. I can well imagine that if William Tell had existed, he would have been an orphan. It is the same in every country. National holidays and remembrance days recall the courage and the faith with which the nation's forbears faced the terrible ordeals of the past. Out of the disaster inflicted by Hitler on France came General De Gaulle's rallying call of the 18th June 1940. André Haynal alludes to it: 'the charismatic leader re-establishes hope'.

Another example, from among so many – and a more peaceful one: when the Russians sent up their first sputnik, there was a real sense of humiliation in the United States, out of which came a great leap forward in American scientific and technological creativity, which led to the landing on the moon. And now that we are faced with the energy crisis are we not seeing how the disappearance of old resources is provoking a feverish search for new sources of energy?

Consider now what has happened to the two most important countries defeated in World War II, Germany and Japan. Their prodigious development is there for all to see, yet you must know that that blaze of creativity was born out of extreme distress. I was in devastated Germany at the time of Dr Erhard's monetary reform, which everyone was saying would finally ruin the country. As for Japan, the miracle was built entirely on the memorable statement by Emperor Hirohito when he announced the surrender: 'We must now accept the unacceptable, and surmount the insurmountable.'

Fortunate is the nation that has such a leader. I rendered him the homage he deserved in my speech in Kobe, when I referred to this memorable appeal to the Japanese nation, to which I applied a maxim that I once heard in one of Dr Biot's sessions on medicine and philosophy, in Lyon: 'A man's value is to be measured not so much by his successes, as by the way he takes his failures.' So intense was the emotion that my interpreter, the eminent Paul Claudel specialist Dr Michio Kurimura, made me repeat it, fearing that he had not understood correctly. But I was quite as moved as he was, having hesitated for a long time before deciding to touch on such a delicate subject. I had foreseen the problem even before I left Geneva. Japan! The name immediately evoked in my mind the thought of the vicious war in the Pacific, which began with the perfidious attack on Pearl Harbour and ended with the dreadful atomic bomb and the humiliating defeat of a proud people. Could I talk about these things in public, I who came from privileged Switzerland which had been spared the experience of war, without offending that well-known Japanese reserve? I took the opportunity of talking about it to my interpreter, and he did not know what to say. Ten days of speeches went by without my daring to say anything about the feelings that the name of Japan inevitably aroused in me.

My friends in Kobe had organized a heart-warming reception for me, at once both glittering and intimate. Speeches and presentations succeeded one another. The title of one of my books had been solemnly and ritually written out in Indian ink, in enormous and impeccable Japanese characters. I felt uncomfortable, and my speech of thanks was perfunctory. But that night I had a dream which revealed my inner conflict.

Had I not come to Japan in order to talk about personal relationships, which have been almost squeezed out in our civilization, not only between doctor and patient, but in all our social contacts? What is it that stands in the way? It is our mental reservations. What is it that makes official or academic speeches so lifeless, like so much empty chatter? It is the fact that we take refuge in objectivity, in generalized ideas, taking great care not to express any feelings of a personal nature. Is it not this, for instance, that raises a wall of silence around a person who is dying? Here was I, being given such a warm, such a personal welcome in Kobe, and yet I just could not express my feelings more simply.

Fortunately we were going on the morrow to visit Nara, the ancient capital, with its huge and impressive Buddha. I took the opportunity of talking over my problem with my interpreter, Miss Ryoko Ito, a specialist in mediaeval French. I really must decide whether or not I should talk about the emotions that had beset me on the subject of Japan during the war. So I suggested to her that we should sit on a little wall at the side of the road, and meditate together in silence for a moment on the problem. Afterwards she said to me, 'The war, the defeat – everyone thinks about it; nobody talks about it. If you do it with tact, with all the love that you bear towards my country, I think that that will be a relief.' That is what I did when we returned to Kobe that evening.

'Everyone thinks about it; nobody talks about it.' Is not that what makes so many people feel so lonely in our present-day society? We are alone with our deepest preoccupations, when we face sickness, old age, death, all our secret deprivations, all the trials of life; we wonder if there is any meaning in it all, or whether it is nothing but a series of blind chances; we are alone too as we meditate upon the strange, disturbing, unjust connection, which I am tackling in this book, between the greatest misfortunes and the most precious blessings. We all have an intuitive and rather disturbing feeling that there is such a connection, at least when we have gained some experience of life; and we are reluctant to talk about it. Is not that the same fear of emotion which was holding me back when I was in Japan?

There is no doubt of it. But I think that there is a deeper and more serious reason for our cautious silence. It is the uneasy feeling, which you have probably had yourself as you have been reading these pages, that in pointing to all the evidence which suggests that human progress is bound up with great individual of historical calamities, we are coming dangerously near to the glorification of suffering, to praising its supposed virtues. Like you, I should find that revolting. Suffering is an evil against which we must fight a battle without quarter. How uneasy we should all feel if the sufferer were to suspect that we thought it was doing him good!

Everyone has a certain intuition about what I have been saying, some awareness of a relationship between the misfortunes which befall mankind, both in the lives of individuals and in those of nations, and the benefits they enjoy, their progress, their creativity. But everyone also feels that the question it raises is a difficult and complex one, and especially dangerous and repellant if it suggests that the relationship is one of cause and effect, or that suffering has didactic value. In the end, would it not weaken our determination to continue the struggle against suffering, if we thought it might be good for people?

I think that is the reason why we so often avoid asking this serious question. We make passing references to it, taking refuge in paradox, witticism, or aphorism, so that the question is not faced squarely, or else we say that 'it is an ill wind that blows nobody any good'; and the proverb allows us to evoke a truth in the form of age-old popular wisdom, without having to think about it or commit ourselves to it as a personal belief. I was talking about this subject recently at the Œcumenical Institute with Madame El Khoury, a writer from Damascus. She at once quoted to me an Arabic proverb (one with which my English readers too will be familiar): 'Necessity is the mother of invention.' But all at once, in the presence of some tragic event, one becomes aware of the seriousness of the problem. Or even in the course of a discussion about suffering.

2

A Blessing in Disguise?

I well remember the day when the seriousness of this problem was first borne in upon me. It was a shock, like a head-on collision, or, if you prefer, like what doctors call a diagnostic 'sign' – that is, a symptom so precise, so clearly localized, that it leaves no doubt about the diagnosis. It was at my own home, the 'Grain de Blé', under the eye of the television camera.

The producer had me sauntering along with a microphone hanging round my neck, beside my cornfield. I was to pick an ear of wheat and toy with it as I spoke. Spoke about what? – About suffering. There and then I said out loud a thing I had been saying to myself for some days on the subject of these studies about orphans. 'Being an orphan? I have always believed it to be the great misfortune of my life, and now I have to admit that it has been the great good fortune of my life!'

A hundredth of a second later I imagined what a sick person would think if he heard me, a doctor, saying such a thing on the TV! I quickly corrected my aim, as you might say; I went on at once to say as I continued my stroll: 'Obviously, I should never tell a patient that he was lucky to be ill.' Fortunately my reflexes were good – but the obvious contradiction left me in confusion. Was suffering not always evil? Could it be a blessing in disguise? Could evil be sometimes evil and sometimes good? It worried me: I had to know!

I had in fact scented the trap a few days before at the end of a conversation with Dr Haynal. I shall come back to it, but first I must tell you about our talk. I had of course written to tell him how moved I had been on reading his admirable essay on deprivation. He had kindly invited me to visit him and his wife, who is also a psychoanalyst. We were in their beautiful sunlit terraced garden, with its view over the fertile plain dominated by the Salève, the whole enchanting countryside of my childhood, for they live only a short distance away from me.

I could see the little village of Bossey, where Jean-Jacques Rousseau, orphaned at an early age, spent two memorable years. And where he too was trapped: the malicious sister of Pastor Lambercier, who had taken him into his home, wrongfully accused him of having broken her comb, and neither she nor the pastor would believe him when he protested his innocence.

The incident had a decisive influence on Rousseau's whole life. He had hoped to find in this new home a little of the maternal tenderness he had been without since his mother's death; particularly since his father had often spoken to him about it in glowing terms. But his father had just been banished from Geneva, and Jean-Jacques found himself orphaned for the second time. And in place of trust he found injustice.

Jean Starobinski shows this clearly in his fine book on Rousseau and the loss of transparency. By transparency he means that quality of openness in human relationships of which Rousseau dreamed, a loyal and confident frankness, free of mental reservations and private judgments, which I call personal relationship. Proof of this is that when I wrote *The Meaning of Persons*, in which I showed how much we suffer in our Western civilization from the lack of this genuine intimacy between persons, readers – both men and women – told me that they had at once noted the similarity between my book and that of Jean Starobinski.

Rousseau was never able to come to terms with this lack of mutual confidence. From then onwards he wandered everywhere in search of a 'place to live', as he put it, denouncing the wickedness of men almost to the point of persecution mania. Finally he sought refuge in Nature, 'in some desert place', as he wrote to Malesherbes, 'where no sign of the hand of man proclaims servitude and domination'. I do not have to remind you of the creativity of Jean-Jacques Rousseau: not only his literary output, but the influence he has exercised on the world. For whoever invokes the democratic ideal, the rights of man, and liberty of conscience, is, without realizing it, the heir of my illustrious fellow-citizen, of his *Discourse on the origin of inequality*, his *Social Contract*, and his famous chapter on religion, the *Confession de foi d'un Vicaire Savoyard*.

I was thinking about all this on the terrace of Dr Haynal's garden. Thinking is not quite the word, unless you can apply it to the still undefined emotional presentiment which, through the free association of ideas, brought into my mind my own experience as an orphan as I contemplated the place where Jean-Jacques Rousseau faced his own experience of dereliction. And so there I was with these two psychoanalysts, in the same position as their patients in their consulting-rooms: in the throes of self-discovery. I was being touched by the magic of personal contact. Perhaps a psychoanalyst or a literary critic could describe the whole of my writings as a long search for maternal tenderness. In fact that is to some extent what Monroe Peaston and Gary Collins have done in their studies of my work.

Meanwhile Dr Haynal and I were talking about the historical enigma which had brought us together. He was surprised at my enthusiasm about his study of deprivation. He pointed out that all he had done was to report the testimony, already well known, of writers and artists, together with facts that everyone knows from his own experience: that it is in trials and suffering that creativity awakes. Shortly afterwards as I was leaving he made the following remark: 'Why is it that in fact we talk so little about all this?'

I replied that I thought it was because for too long we have made the mistake of looking on suffering as a good thing. In the Middle Ages especially it was a favourite theme. That was the trap into which I myself had fallen when I spoke in front of the television camera about my good luck in having been an orphan – as if deprivation could ever be a blessing! Then, at the Renaissance, they had had enough of suffering, and we have seen how much they suffered at that time. They began to study nature in order the better to be able to combat suffering. A complete revolution took place in the field of values: the cult of self-denial was replaced by that of self-assertion; preoccupation with a future life in heaven by concern for life on earth now; obsession with sin by the quest for progress; worship of age by the cult of youth and strength; the impenetrable mystery of the world by exact scientific knowledge; the obscurity of metaphysics by the clarity of experimental physics.

The whole prodigious development of science and technology results from this inversion of values. The movement passes through the century of the Enlightenment, and then through the philosophy of positivism, which is still that of most doctors, as Gusdorf has shown in his *Dialogue avec le médecin*. But it manifests itself also in industrialization, with its augmentation of production, in urbanization – is it not in order to enjoy the resources of the city that the peasant leaves his land? – in the consumer society and its mad insistence on economic growth. It is no part of my purpose to belittle the incomparable benefits that this has brought at least to us who live in the rich countries. To us the last few centuries appear as a vast and victorious campaign against material deprivation. It is when we come to the trials and tribulations of life, to disease and death, that we see that spiritual deprivation, however, has increased.

You know well that the movement to which I refer has culminated in the great master-critics – Glucksmann's 'Masterminds': Nietzsche, Marx, Freud – in the dechristianization of the West, in the drying up of the inner life and of piety, in the loss of a sense of the meaning of life, in greater distress in face of suffering and death, in Riesman's 'solitary crowd', and in the tedium of life in industrialized societies, of which Ricoeur speaks.

There is, then, a great danger in religious circles, in the heat of controversy, of clinging to the idea that there is some virtue in suffering and deprivation which is not appreciated by this material world in its prosperity and its glorification of health, wealth, and success. As if there were two camps, that of the unbelievers who struggle desperately against deprivation of all kinds, and that of the believers who preach renunciation. The notion that there is some virtue in suffering did not die with the Middle Ages. I have seen many people, often from religious families, who have still retained from their childhood this idea of the value of suffering, and of a terrible God who uses it to chastise mankind for its own good. Even atheists often have some vague idea of a law of nature or fate which condemns man to suffer in order to achieve progress.

Of course I am not intending here to tackle the whole problem of the origin of evil, which no philosopher has ever been able to solve. I am no more than a practitioner who observes men and their reactions to the troublesome ups and downs of life in order to understand and help them. When we are young, good and evil seem quite distinct from each other. Parents and teachers do all they can to persuade the young of this. Legends and fairy-tales too always make a clear distinction between the virtuous folk and the wicked ogre who is the incarnation of all evil.

Eventually we lose our illusions and discover that evil is everywhere, even insinuating itself into our noblest actions. How often does the hidden selfishness of love turn itself into tyranny; how much pride there can be in 'good works'; how much hate in the most altruistic political and social campaigns; how much vanity in drawing-room conversations and academic debates – and in fact in all men's actions: are not those whom we see as presumptuous simply the ones who find it harder to hide their vanity? And if I confess that I too am vain, am I not still doing so out of vanity?

All this has its funny side, and that is the line taken by the cartoonists, whose work I greatly enjoy, and who find this universal hypocrisy an inexhaustible mine for their humour. But laughter can slide into bitter and destructive cynicism. One's laughter dies away when one thinks of all the suffering that these unconscious faults can cause.

Jesus was able to look into this unconscious region of men's minds. He sternly denounced the sin of the 'righteous', as Ricoeur points out – the sin which proceeds from the depths of the heart, despite outward appearances of virtue. At this point the gospel is in line with modern psychology. As soon as we investigate the motivation of our thoughts and actions we see that the best and the worst are as inextricably mixed together as are the oxygen and the nitrogen in the air we breathe. I have seen many people quite overwhelmed by this discovery, as their experience of life or psychological analysis brought them to maturity, so that they looked back with a certain nostalgia to the simplicity of their childhood, when good and evil were clearly distinguishable from each other.

The fact is that evil is everywhere mixed with good. The

Bible proclaims the fact and our experience confirms it. Since I have really understood this, I am no longer astonished that there is so much evil in the world – as the newspapers, as well as the countless confidences of my patients, keep telling me. Jesus referred to the mixture in his parable of the wheat and the tares, which it was impossible to sort out before the harvest. And yet no confusion is possible between good and evil. The good grain was sown by God; as for the tares, they were the work of 'some enemy' (Matt. 13.28). None of the ears of wheat has come from a seed of tares, and none of the tares has grown from a grain of wheat. There is a mixture, but no confusion. Good is the cause of good, and evil causes evil. Evil cannot be the cause of good.

What then of the relationship that exists between deprivation and suffering, and creativity – apparently between evil and good? But relationship is not the same as cause. You remember Dr Haynal's remark which I quoted: 'There is a relationship between the processes of bereavement, loss, deprivation, and creativity.' He carefully refrains from saying that it is a relationship of cause and effect. The person matures, develops, becomes more creative, not because of the deprivation in itself, but through his own active response to misfortune, through the struggle to come to terms with it and morally to overcome it – even if in spite of everything there is no cure. My good luck was not in being an orphan, but that I was helped to overcome the consequences of that particular deprivation.

You are well aware of this, and so was I, but it took the incident on television to show me the importance of the distinction. That was the trap – to confuse relationship with cause, and hence to say that suffering is good for one. The distinction is a subtle one, of course, but it is vital. You remember the former patient whom I met in the street, and who told me that with hindsight, and at this distance of time, he looked upon the period of his illness as one of the most fruitful in his life. That does not mean that sickness had been the cause of growth, but rather its occasion. The growth had resulted from his own personal reaction to his misfortune. He could equally well have regressed, passively allowing himself to go under.

Good and evil, in the moral sense, do not reside in things, but always in persons. Things and events, whether fortunate or unfortunate, are simply what they are, morally neutral. What matters is the way we react to them. Only rarely are we the masters of events, but (along with those who help us) we are responsible for our reactions. I always remember what my wife said when she tripped and fell over the dog, and broke her leg. I told her that her leg was fractured and that she would have to go into hospital. She replied, 'So many people have to go to hospital; it's only right that for once it should be my turn!' As for the dog, he suffered from a guilt neurosis which paralysed his back legs, and he dragged himself about on his belly, using only his front legs. At the very moment when my wife returned home he began to frolic about again.

Events give us pain or joy, but our growth is determined by our personal response to both, by our inner attitude. This attitude, of course, is already itself the fruit of our whole previous growth. And at each stage in the long chain of experiences that makes up a life, innumerable factors enter into the reckoning; physical, psychological, and social factors, but also ethical and spiritual ones. I am not going to say here all that there is to be said on the great and controversial problem of free will. But it is already involved when we talk of the way we react to events – the question is, are we free at that point, or not?

Ferdinand Gonseth had already demonstrated, in his book on determinism and free will, that it was impossible honestly to eliminate either of the two apparently contradictory theses, and that for a real understanding of man a synthesis must be found, whatever the difficulty. Against the scientist who can see nothing but the rigorous determinism of causality, he said, stands the 'individualist' who recognizes his responsibility for the choices he makes, for his convictions and his actions. He is a disturbing embarrassment to the scientist who, secure in his closed system of thought, is yet unable either to gainsay him or to silence him.

The argument has been taken up now by Dr Jacques Sarano in his book *L'homme double*. In each one of us there are two contradictory men: the critical man and the ethical man. The critical man is the man of objectivity, who recognizes only an inexorable chain of cause and effect, or even, nowadays, the finalism of the new idea of genetic programming, which is just as inexorable. The ethical man judges himself as a responsible subject. So Sarano quotes Vergès, who 'eliminates the ethical man in favour of the critical man, in the name of philosophical rationality'. Obviously that is rather too easy a way of solving the contradiction! 'But will it do,' Sarano asks, 'to dismiss the problem by rejecting free will and so washing one's hands of it? . . . Is not philosophical thought, or simply human thought, bound to wrestle with the enigma of man and his fundamental contradiction? In what way is ethical affirmation any less "philosophical" than critical evidence?'

Of course there are automatisms. If you belong to the school of Pavlov, you see the part played by conditioning, as evidenced by his experiments with the dog. It is true so far as it goes, but it is not the whole story, because we are men who ask ourselves questions about the meaning of life, which the dog does not do. If you are a psychoanalyst you see the part played by unconscious impulses in the determination of a repetitive behaviour pattern. That is also true, but again it is not the whole story, because we are men with a conscious life, with convictions and a sense of values. At this point we ought to quote Charles Odier, with his *Deux sources, consciente et inconsciente, de la vie morale*. If there are values which are no more than functions of conditioning or of our unconscious impulses, there are also authentic values to which we adhere of our own free will.

There is constant interplay among all these factors. But the remarkable thing is that the study of automatic mechanisms, which are accessible to science, helps us constantly to revise our scale of values so as to be better able to distinguish the true values and to respond to them in our behaviour. And so fortunate and unfortunate events – and especially the tragic events, the deprivations – are not the cause of our growth, but occasions for the manifestation through the way we react to them of our fundamental attitude. What Gonseth calls the individualist, is in my view what Sarano calls the 'affirmation of the self'. By definition science recognizes only objects. It puts the subject in parenthesis. However long the parenthesis is, it must in the end be closed, and then one comes back to the self, our personal manner of responding to events.

What is wrong here is the old Latin tag: *Post hoc, ergo propter hoc* ('After this, therefore on account of this'). There is a relationship, but it is one of succession, not of cause. Fine weather always follows bad weather, but that does not mean that it is caused by it. Much more, if on delving into the past lives of the great creative figures of history, one almost always finds great misfortunes, that is a long way from saying that, conversely, every misfortune is succeeded by a creative renewal.

For the few hundreds of orphans listed by Rentchnick who have made a name for themselves in history, there are millions whom deprivation in childhood has handicapped for life. This objection had not escaped him, and in his article he wrote that orphans make good only 'in so far as they have the necessary intellectual and temperamental equipment'. It is quite probable that the famous men he cites were endowed with an exceptional genetic code. But for the majority, not only of orphans but of all those who suffer misfortune, their reaction depends, I think, much more on the help they receive from others than on their hereditary disposition.

The whole of my career has taught me, in fact, how difficult it is for anyone on his own, without outside help, to overcome the consequences of any serious moral trauma. I say my career, but I might also say my own personal experience. Quite frankly, I do not reckon that I was endowed with unusual unconscious will to power, as I was ready to admit on reading my colleague's article. On the other hand, I cannot measure how much I owe to all who came to my aid. First an uncle and aunt who received me with affection into their home, gave me material security and a liberal education, religious instruction and ideals of loyalty and service, and paid for the medical studies which I had chosen.

Then my classics teacher who invited me to his house, took an interest in me not only as a pupil but as a person, which made me into a person, initiated me into intellectual argument and social action. Next, wonderful friendships, the experiences I had in the Red Cross and in the church, and during the early years of my career as a general practitioner. Finally, at the age of thirty-four, the great turning-point in my life in the Oxford Group, a movement which put the accent on personal contact and complete openness between individuals about our problems and our emotions, and on listening for God, and concrete obedience to his will for us in our personal, family, and professional lives. It transformed my relationship with my sons, with my friends and my patients, and forged firm friendships with so many of them, but especially with my wife, Nelly, who became my partner in the search for God, my confidant and my confessor.

In all this I perceive the grace of God. It was he who came
to my aid by making so many people the instruments of his
love. Long ago I gave a lecture in Strasbourg. On that occasion
the Community of Deaconesses invited me to a meal. On my
arrival the Superior informed me that it was their custom that
one of them should read a verse from the Bible and comment
briefly upon it, and she asked me if I would do this. A liturgical
calendar indicated the verse for the day. It was 'I will not leave
you orphans' (John 14.18). Think how appropriate that was!
I was able quite simply to say, 'That saying came true for me.' I
had lost one father and mother, and God gave me many, without any of them usurping my parents' place. And so many
brothers and sisters, and spiritual children.

I am telling all this in broad outline, where small details
would be more vivid: an elderly cousin who used to invite me
affectionately to her home. An old friend of my father's who
used to talk to me about him. I used to go and see him in the
Rue de l'Evêché in the old town, where there was a fine view
of the harbour. He was a historian, and told me that he worked
every night until four o'clock in the morning, and that impressed me because I had reluctantly to go early to bed. He
showed me his enormous card-index of references, and that is
no doubt why I have kept one myself throughout my life. I feel
the truth of the biblical promises of divine blessing on the
descendants of pious and faithful ancestors, and how I have
been supported by the prayers of my parents and of those who
loved them. Remember that I was five when my mother died:
though all memory of her caresses has gone, repressed into my
unconscious, I was certainly not deprived of them in those
early years of my life when they were most necessary.

Here I am, recording my privileges, everything that I have
not been deprived of! Perhaps you are smiling – mocking me
a little for writing like that in a book on deprivation! But this

time it is not a contradiction. It is complementary. It is obvious that in all our lives there is a mixture of privileges and deprivations, and it is hard to talk about them both at the same time. Hard too to weigh them up. Are there not wretched little waifs who once experienced a maternal tenderness which many a rich child has never known at all? And if they develop into healthy, rounded personalities, may that not be due to the psychological stamina which that tenderness gave them, as much as to the fact that they are orphans? It is possible to draw up statistics about orphans, but not about emotional deprivation.

As I said, in the life of each of us there is a mixture of privileges and deprivations. The proportions of each are variable, and impossible to quantify. Deprivations without the aid of love spell catastrophe. But privileges without much in the way of deprivations mean retrogression. What bears fruit is in fact the mixture of both; just as the most favourable climate is the one in which good weather alternates with bad. André Missenard points out that the most propitious regions for the development of civilization are those with the greatest contrast between the heat of summer and the cold of winter. For the human personality the decisive factor in making deprivation bear fruit is love. Love, one might say, changes the sign of deprivation from minus to plus. Without love, deprivation has a negative coefficient. Love applies a positive coefficient.

That is what happened to me. It was the genuine and quite personal love of my adoptive family, my classics master, my wife, of lots of other people and above all of my friends in the Oxford Group Movement that changed my destiny and liberated me from the handicap of being an orphan. The fourteen years I spent as an activist in the Movement were for me a veritable school of love. I left it when it changed its character under the leadership of its founder, Dr Frank Buchman, and became Moral Rearmament. From then on it saw itself as a Christian ideology to be set against other ideologies, which is not my scene – I am concerned with the individual person and the problems peculiar to it.

During the Oxford Group period, however, it did concern itself with my problems. In the Movement I was able to open my heart to friends on the subject of my life, my feelings, my fears, and to talk about the things I was ashamed of and the things I longed for. Though I did not realize it at the time, it was a real psychological treatment for me. Indeed, apart from the religious experience involved, namely the experience of the grace of God, of his nearness to me in meditation, and of brotherly love, there was in it everything that is characteristic of psychoanalysis: catharsis, emotional discharge, awareness, and transference. Then other people in their turn came to me and opened their hearts. I was becoming something of a psychoanalyst.

I could have gone the whole way. I asked myself seriously, and some of my colleagues also put it to me, whether I wanted to take up psychiatry. I should have had to devote two years to specialist studies in the subject, and to perform a dialectical analysis. Ought I to take the plunge? Twice over I turned to friends for advice: first to Dr Alphonse Maeder, one of the very first psychoanalysts, since he was with C. G. Jung when together they made their first memorable visit to Freud in Vienna. A few years later I approached Dr Théo Bovet, who had made both a Freudian and a Jungian analysis.

Each of them replied in the negative to my question; and both used, literally, and without collusion, the same words: 'We are not short of good psychoanalysts, there are plenty of them; but we have only one Paul Tournier.' That obviously meant that in their view I had to follow my own personal vocation, and attempt a synthesis between psychology and classical medicine – and even religious belief. The danger for the specialist is that of interpreting everything in accordance with the theory he has received from his teacher. A synthesis will be achieved only if one is free from all dogmatic prejudice. So there, I did not become a psychoanalyst; I opted for the medicine of the person, the non-specialized attitude *par excellence*, which seeks to understand man as a whole – the importance of the body, which the psychologist is in danger of neglecting, the importance of the psyche, which the organicist is in danger of forgetting, and the importance of religious faith, which may escape the doctor who confines himself exclusively to science.

So, for forty years now, in all my books, I have been tramping regardless over all the barriers which the analytical spirit of our civilization has carefully been erecting between the various disciplines; not only the medicine of the body, genetics, and psychology, but also sociology, education, economics, history, literature, theology, and philosophy. Of course I lack competence in each of these individual disciplines, and the experts find it easy to denounce my mistakes and see me as a perpetual heretic.

But is it not a misfortune for our civilization to have this plethora of eminent specialists, each in his watertight compartment? I observe it in the doctors whom I call together. Coming away from the conference-hall after a fine address by a psychoanalyst, I meet a surgeon and say to him, 'That was remarkable, wasn't it?' He replies, 'I didn't understand a single word.'

It is just as true in other spheres. I am at present reading Maurice Guernier's report to the famous Club of Rome. He points out that the problem of the Third World – the undoubted key to the economic problems of our time – will remain insoluble so long as it is debated in conference after conference only by expert economists obsessed by the GNP as the sole measure of development. 'The most striking thing in the politics of the whole of the Third World,' he writes, 'is the absence of creativity, the absence of creative imagination. Everything is copied from the Old World. Nothing is original, nothing is natural, nothing is young.' We come back, as you see, to our problem of creativity. Is there going to be an awakening of creativity in the present crisis?

The fact is that we find on the world scale the same thing that so profoundly moves me, as a doctor, in all those who come to me for help. As we have clearly seen, suffering is never beneficial in itself, and must always be fought against. What counts is the way a person reacts in face of suffering. That is the real test of the person: what is our personal attitude to life and its changes and chances. Here is a man, sick or in the grip of some tragedy, who confides in me: what is he going to make of the grievous blow that has struck him? What is his personal reaction going to be? A positive, active, creative reaction which will develop his person, or a negative one that will stunt it? As we saw in the case of the orphans, one will go on to play an important part in history; another will be a permanent failure. The right help given at the right moment may determine the course of a whole life.

It is like a game of chess, in which a single weak move can compromise the whole game. Especially when one considers the 'snowball effect': every courageous reaction is bracing, it renews hope and makes fresh victories easier; and every defeat makes way for further withdrawals. It is like a watershed. We think of it as being along the mountain-tops, but it can be in the plain. On the Swiss plateau there is a spot amusingly called the 'Middle of the World', because of two drops of rain falling side by side there, one will make its way to the North Sea via the Rhine, and the other to the Mediterranean via the Rhone.

Another analogy which my patients often employ is that of

the tunnel: one can get out by going either forward or backward. And Dr Haynal, writing of the artist hit by misfortune, says that he must 'transform it creatively or go under'. One is reminded of Goethe and the masterpiece he wrote in the midst of disappointment in love.

Of course every moment in life is a challenge, but there are times – the times of life's greatest trials – when the challenge suddenly becomes more intense, more imperiously urgent. For a number of years I took part in an anthropological research group organized in Strasbourg by a Dutch colleague, Dr De Moll van Otterloo. Among other projects, Paul Ricoeur and I were asked to write a book together on 'man in crisis situations', because it is then that man reveals what he is. However, the departure of Paul Ricoeur for the Sorbonne, summoned by other concerns, cut our plans short.

But now I find myself considering once again the decisive importance of the response of any man to serious misfortune. It never leaves him exactly as he was before. Much will depend on those who have helped him to choose courage. The powerful machine of technological medicine tends rather to turn him into a passive object undergoing treatment in which he takes no part. He waits to be healed by it, and feels that only after that will he take on responsibility for himself once more. The doctor, for his part, is only too ready to believe that he is fulfilling his whole task in working for the cure, and sustaining the patient's confidence in it.

3

Win or Lose?

So there is always a double hazard: will he recover or not? Will
he grow under misfortune or not? And if there is a double risk
for the patient, there is a double task for the doctor: to work
towards healing, and to help the patient to make, in Pascal's
words, good use of his sickness. What gives our vocation as
doctors a humanist significance is precisely the fact that we are
always meeting people in 'crisis situations', at the moment when
disease or some other misfortune has suddenly interrupted the
routine of their lives and brought them face to face with their
destiny.

They are thinking of it, more or less consciously, much more
frequently than we suspect. They are not stupid! Even in the
case of some slight everyday disease – and it is because it is
slight that they dare allude to it – at the end of the consultation,
as they are leaving, they ask their question, half joking: 'Well,
doctor, is it serious?' Which means, 'Am I in danger of dying,
and what would be the meaning of my life if I died?'

People do not realize the extent to which the routine of active
life in our smooth-running and tyrannical civilization cuts them
off from what is essential. The thing that will stimulate their
personal maturation is this brutal confrontation with the existential problems they have managed to forget. It is easy to talk
of scientific data, laboratory tests, and X-rays – in reality a sort
of complicity of silence! Naturally I am not suggesting long

philosophical discussions at such a moment; a simple gesture, a glance or a word will suffice to make the patient feel that these technological details are not the only questions that arise.

The doctor therefore has two tasks. One is pressing, immediate: his scientific, technological task. The other is helping his patient to profit from his sickness to the benefit of his personal development. It is a long-term task, in which he must recognize that growth takes time. In distinguishing these two tasks I am not suggesting that they are either mutually exclusive or of equal importance. The difference between them is fundamental: the doctor alone is responsible for the fulfilment of his scientific task, since that is what he is qualified for; whereas anyone can help a patient in his personal development.

You will have seen the truth of this from the list of those to whom I owe my own rescue: there was hardly a doctor among them. There was one, however – my own GP, Dr Chenevière, when I was a child. I well remember, at the time when I felt that I did not matter to anybody, the exceptional impression made on me by that man, with all the prestige he had in my eyes, simply because he cared personally about me. That was no doubt one of the reasons for my choice of a medical vocation. I say that the doctor has an existential task, because at this critical moment in the life of the patient he finds himself in a privileged and intimate relationship with him, entrusted with his confidence, and better placed than anyone else to understand and help him; and also because the way the patient reacts will affect the cure, and that reaction depends very largely upon the quality of his relationship with his doctor.

The doctor's scientific task nevertheless remains of prime importance, and its moral and spiritual implications can in no way excuse a lack of professional expertise. It was Pastor Bernard Martin, whose books on spiritual healing are well known, who wrote: 'If I can choose between a very humane but poorly qualified doctor, and one who is cold but well qualified, I shall choose the second.' All who are ill will agree with him. They have but one desire – to get well. And that is the answer I have always given to students who have come to ask my advice on how to prepare themselves for the medicine of the person: 'Begin by taking your studies at the Medical School as seriously as possible.'

But even if the patient is concerned only with getting better, and has no thought for his evolution as a person, that evolution will take place, for better or for worse, without his realizing it. He will become aware of it later. And the change, as we have seen, will have been occasioned by the illness.

The same applies to any other situation of deprivation – bereavement, infirmity, marital conflict; or the suffering of a dear one, which, as André Maurois has pointed out, is harder to bear than our own. The patient who consults us is also concerned only to find relief in his trouble, a cure for his depression, generally without suspecting that this will have an effect on his evolution as a person. I can prescribe drugs for him, listen to him sympathetically, but that is not enough.

Try for once, my dear colleague, to step out of your scientific objectivity, and talk to him in a personal manner, talk to him about the darkest hours of your own life, the long struggle you had, your rebellions, and those who helped you to win through. You will have brought together the two tasks I spoke of, without having betrayed the first of them. And see how necessary it is to bring them together, for example in the case of a marital conflict, which always derives, as you know, from lack of maturity in one or both of the spouses, and from the absence of real dialogue between them.

So the doctor alone is responsible for his scientific task. He cannot in conscience avoid the second, but there he is no longer alone; he shares it with everyone else. And a good thing, too! Who does not see, for example, that there will never be enough psychotherapists to cope with the enormous tide of psychological troubles that has been flowing for the last hundred years in our Western civilization, to say nothing of the violence, drug-addiction, divorce, and suicide? That is because it arises from the faults in our civilization, of which it is a symptom, and it will begin to recede only when far-reaching changes take place in our society. And that is the task, not of specialists, but of all of us.

I come back to the Report by Maurice Guernier to the Club of Rome to which I referred just now. He points out that the problem of the Third World will remain insoluble so long as it is discussed only by the economists in their innumerable conferences of experts, because there are too many non-economic factors which escape them – political, psychological, ethnological, cultural, demographical, and ethical. He is an economist himself, and this gives his Report its authority. He is not trying to avoid his task, therefore, but rather to share it, to enlarge it into a collaboration among specialists of various disciplines, which is indeed the purpose of the Club of Rome.

Reading it I was reminded of Clémenceau's famous remark: 'War is too serious a matter to be left to the military.' Similarly, I might say that the economic crisis is too serious a matter to be left to the economists. And again, man's health – not only the prevention of epidemics, or organ transplants, but also the promotion of man's physical, psychological, and social welfare as defined by the WHO – is too serious a matter to be left to doctors alone. I might add morality, philosophy, theology, sociology . . . The misfortune of our time, as I see clearly in medicine, is not the specialization which has brought so much progress, but the fact that the specialists work in ever more water-tight compartments.

The medicine of the person is not one more specialism, in preparation for which psychology, sociology, theology, and philosophy would have to be added to our training curricula. It is, in the spirit of the Club of Rome, a meeting-place of specialists who learn through their communication together that in the actual accomplishment of their specific scientific task, they are already assuming responsibility for the second task of medicine, namely that of helping men and women not only to recover from their ills, but to learn something from the experience in order to grow and to live better lives.

To my organicist colleagues, who modestly refuse to follow me outside the strict frontiers of scientific objectivity, I like to say that they are already exerting a powerful subjective moral influence through the very zeal with which they carry out their technological task. It makes an important contribution to the personal development of the patient. The careful attention he receives will be a most important factor to help him on his long journey from rejection to acceptance. What is sometimes needed is a little more real dialogue between doctor and patient, even if it is only about the details of his treatment.

Why, then, refuse to pay attention also to the spiritual evolution of the patient and to recognize that it has an important part to play in the success of the treatment? Why opt out when the patient attempts to unburden himself about his intimate and even his religious preoccupations? There are plenty of opportunities if you are not afraid to take them. Even the most confirmed non-believer will exclaim: 'What have I done for God to let this happen to me?' Why not reply? The problem of suffering is a serious one, as we have seen; everybody thinks about it. Why turn the patient over to some psychiatrist or clergyman whom he does not know? It is to you that he has entrusted his life; he expects everything from you, and it is with you, too, that he would like to have an honest dialogue.

Once, in a conference of American general practitioners I used an expression they know well: 'Why not "do it yourself"?', I asked them.

Finally, as we all know, science can assert what it can prove by experiment or by calculation, but it is not at liberty to deny what lies outside the scope of its methods. Healing always takes place through the medium of phenomena which are biological – that is to say, physiological, which is to say, chemical. Now, the speed of a chemical reaction is doubled with each rise in temperature of four degrees, which involves a geometrical progression in its rate of acceleration. You know the fantastic consequences of such progressions, as illustrated by the old story of the grain of wheat placed on one square of a chessboard.

There is no reason to suppose that a spiritual energy which we cannot measure might not be capable of causing an acceleration analogous with that due to temperature. This could be the explanation of certain of the cures performed by Jesus (there were some, such as the healing of a blind man, and that of a number of lepers – Mark 8.22 – which were not instantaneous), as well as others that have occurred throughout history, and are still observable in the Charismatic Movement. This would be what was termed bio-radiant energy by Dr Francesco Racanelli, who was a faith-healer before becoming a doctor.

One further remark on this subject. The body is an organism, a whole whose parts are strictly dependent on each other and upon the whole. Science, however, being analytical, excels in the study of the parts, but is powerless to grasp the whole – the person. Thus doctors seek to heal the whole by healing the parts, whereas Jesus, it seems, healed the parts by healing the whole.

Furthermore, the healing at which you aim has for the patient a magical glamour, as if it would solve all his problems at a stroke. But it is much more complex than he supposes, as Dr Pierre Granjon has pointed out in his book on the nature of healing. It would often be worth talking a little more about it, in order to exorcize these magical notions. The price of healing may be that the individual is permanently disabled, or left with after-effects that will change his life completely.

Doctors know that apart from a few surgical cases – and that is what makes surgery attractive – this whole question of healing is not one of black and white, but rather of many shades of grey. This is especially true in psychology, in which the success of the treatment consists much more in unmasking unconscious impulses in order to be able courageously to master them, than in being simply freed from them. Last winter in the deep snows of the Jura Mountains there took place a friendly gathering of doctors practising the medicine of the person in the Canton of Neuchâtel. Dr Rüedi, the medical director of the Hôpital des Cadolles, who presided, proposed to us a common theme: 'Living with our complexes, for want of resolving them'. I thought at once of my great shyness, which I have never been able to overcome, and which I should once again have to face in order to admit it!

In the case of heart disease, hypertension, diabetes, arthritis, and so many other complaints, healing can only be in the form of remission from an acute episode, and will still leave after-effects with which the patient will have to come to terms, like the neurotic with his complexes, to which Dr Rüedi was referring. And then there are those implacable diseases from which, humanly speaking, there is no reasonable hope of recovery.

Well, I must admit that when I began to prepare this book, noting down my random ideas, each on a separate slip of paper, to be set in order later like the pieces in a puzzle, thinking about this double task of the doctor I wrote on one of the slips: 'If there is no longer any chance of a cure, there is still the chance of growing, of making a success of life.' When, later on, I re-read what I had written there, I exclaimed aloud, 'How awful!'

We must be careful when speaking or writing not to be carried away by the magic of words, so that we over-state our case! It is like the incident of my TV interview which I related earlier; it lends itself to serious misunderstanding. In the first place, no one makes a success of his life. Even our most decisive experiences have their limitations. The greatest of all – personal encounter with God in Jesus Christ – is but a payment on account, according to St Paul (II Cor. 5.5), for, as he says, 'We must be content to hope that we shall be saved' (Rom. 8.24). Furthermore, it is absurd to put the great struggle to preserve life side by side with personal development, as if the latter could ever compensate for failure in the former.

Perhaps what is wrong is this notion of the two-fold task of the doctor. There is no difficulty over his scientific task. But the other, which I describe as human or existential, is not a matter of 'developing someone'. Nobody develops anybody else! Our patients develop themselves by themselves, to the extent that they profit from the experiences through which they live. That is the great lesson which the psychoanalysts have taught us. All they have done is to apply to psychology the great principle of the whole of medicine already formulated by Hippocrates, namely reliance on Nature. Reliance on Nature and reliance on God are the same thing, since he is the creator of Nature, he is concealed in it and reveals himself in it as he does in the supernatural world of the spirit. It is wrong-headed to make the distinction we do between supernatural and natural healing. All healing, and all personal growth, come from God.

Here again modern psychology is in complete accord with the gospel. What are the models to which Jesus points us? The birds in the sky and the flowers in the fields, which God feeds and clothes (Matt. 6.26,28); or again, little children (Matt. 18.3). He inveighs against the Pharisees who take so much trouble to achieve perfection. One of them he contrasts with the poor woman sobbing at his feet (Luke 7.44). Like all those people who weep in our consulting rooms and in their distress achieve personal growth without realizing it, and without our doing anything at all.

So our second task as doctors is not to bring about the personal development of our patients, nor to convert them to our own beliefs, nor even to preach to them. If you do that, my dear colleague, it is as a witness to Jesus and not as a doctor, as I may do with anyone at all. My task as a doctor is to listen to my patient, to try to understand him, to give him a chance to say what he wants to say, to take seriously the questions that are in his mind amid the anxiety of what he is going through, to be really ready to talk with him, most importantly of all if he is facing the greatest of all the trials of life – the conscious descent towards death, the supreme deprivation.

In this last respect great progress has been made since I was a student. Then we simply had to take refuge in lies. It was above all in the USA that courageous and compassionate doctors decided to take their task to its logical conclusion, and systematically to engage in dialogue with those for whom there was no cure. You will have read of the overwhelming experience it turned out to be for them, the extraordinary personal growth they witnessed in larger numbers of patients, and which Frances Horn described to us in a talk she gave at one of our conferences on the medicine of the person.

Let us return, however, to everyday medicine, to the two things that are in the balance in every illness; the possibility of healing, and the possibility of personal growth, of which it may be the occasion. The patient, generally speaking, thinks only of healing, and that is normal. But it seems to me that the study which we are pursuing in this book may encourage the doctor, and possibly the family and friends of the patient, to look further; and that this wider perspective will give his mission a new and exciting dimension. He will see something more than a case that raises scientific questions.

That is the attitude of faith, which waits upon what God may do for both the healing and the growth of the person. For the patient the doctor represents his hope of being healed. If the doctor is imbued with a second hope, the support he gives his patient will be greater still, even if he does not voice it. His concern for the moment is the fight against the disease. If he were to talk about the distant future the patient would feel he was not paying attention to his healing task, that he was being forsaken. To carry on the fight, doctor and patient must be together in the hour of battle. The doctor is like my farmer sowing his corn: he too is looking to the future, thinking of the harvest. He is paying attention to the task of the moment, but he is inspired by a more distant vision.

This time-lag is very important for the problem with which we are concerned in this book. I must tell you now how it was that this suddenly struck me. It was in Coventry, in the course of our thirty-second session on the medicine of the person, which was very well organized this year by our British colleagues. I shall not, of course, try to tell you all about it – you need to take part in one of our meetings in order to discover its creative originality. I record only certain things that are relevant to our subject.

The theme was 'loneliness' – deprivation *par excellence*, characteristic of our modern civilization, and an appropriate theme for doctors engaged in the medicine of the person: think of all those patients who consult their GPs about symptoms of depression, exhaustion, back pains, insomnia, cardiac and digestive troubles, and many more, their real sickness being loneliness. Those who suffer from loneliness find it very hard to put into words. They even hide it as if they were ashamed of it. Dr Heinrich Huebschmann of Heidelberg was there. I am fond of quoting a memorable remark of his: 'When the spirit is silent, the body cries out.' The practitioner of the medicine of the person is able to discern the hidden suffering. Without in any way disregarding the external factors which contribute to loneliness, since it is the scourge of our society, we were able to see that its victims always bear some responsibility for it themselves; so that progress in their own personal development is necessary if they are to be healed.

Dr Richard Sosnowski of Charleston, S. Carolina, leading us in Bible study, spoke of the two solitudes of Jesus: that at the beginning of his ministry, in the temptation in the wilderness (Luke 4). That was a loneliness that was sought, a willing acceptance of the call of the Spirit, the meditation which is so little practised in our restless modern world, and which nevertheless is such a help towards self-discovery and the realization of a personal vocation. And then at the end of his ministry the awful loneliness in Gethsemane (Matt. 26.36) and on the cross, a solitude that was suffered, compounded by betrayal and abandonment by his friends who did not understand what was happening, and even by doubt about the faithfulness of his Father (Matt. 27.46).

We talked at length about the loneliness of pioneers, for example, of those who leave the beaten track and resist the pressures of social conformity. They are the leaven of creativity in society, but inevitably isolated from it. That was the sort of loneliness I myself experienced for three years when I decided to give a new direction to my career, which my best friends failed to understand until my first book was published. But we also talked too much, in an over-simplified fashion, of good and bad loneliness, as if they were always distinct.

At one point, however, Monique Kressmann, the wife of a French doctor, came to the rostrum to announce in tones that carried conviction: 'I am sure that there are not two kinds of loneliness, good and bad, but one.' We all looked at one another in surprise. In order to explain what she meant, Monique told of something that had happened several years before. I spoke up, asking if she could give us a more up-to-date example. Then she began courageously to tell us about a stormy argument she had had with her husband shortly before coming to Coventry – she told the story as only a woman can!

You are perhaps thinking that I exaggerate when I say 'only a woman'. It is scarcely exaggeration! Take, for instance, another couple – this time a husband and wife in conflict – who came to consult me. They told me that the very day before they had had a frightful row. I asked the husband what the argument had been about. He was at a loss for words, unable to tell me; he simply could not remember what they had quarrelled over nor what they had said to each other. He was obviously embarrassed, as he was an intelligent businessman accustomed to remembering things without difficulty.

When I questioned the wife, however, she was able to repeat for me, word for word, everything they had said to each other as if she had recorded it on tape! The acid remark made by her husband which had hurt her like a blow in the face, the cruel reply she had thrown back at him, the torrent of reproaches that that had provoked, and so on. Why this contrast between them? It is because a man is sensitive to intellectual abstractions, and a woman to concrete realities; a man expresses ideas, and a woman feelings. Had it been a discussion about ideas, the husband would have been able to give a clear and ordered account of it, to analyse the arguments as if he were setting it all out in an academic lecture. But there had been no academic debate; only an emotional explosion.

It is not for me, of course, to tell you what Monique Kressmann said; but it was so alive, so concrete, so full of details in which each of us recognized himself, that she had us all laughing out loud. We were the readier to laugh because we were all so fond of the Kressmanns – a delightful, distinguished, and closely-united pair, an example even to us of the perfect spiritual communion that can be established between a husband and wife of different religious denominations.

Monique exclaimed, 'You laugh, you are all laughing, and I can laugh with you now! But I can assure you that I wasn't laughing then. I felt desperately lonely, misunderstood by my husband, everything collapsing round me. Loneliness is always a terrible thing; it is only afterwards that you can see things differently.'

It occurred to me that the situation could be compared to the way the whistle of a train changes its pitch at the precise moment when it passes us, because at first the speed of the train towards us raises the perceived frequency of the sound waves, and then as it recedes the frequency is lowered. In the same way our view of events can change according to whether they are threatening us, are with us in the present, or belong to the past. It is not the events that change, but our perception of them. It is only afterwards that the unhappiest experiences may appear to have been good for us.

It is afterwards that we talk of the creativity of a Descartes. We make a very rapid jump from the little one-year-old orphan to the fully mature man. In accordance with Dr Rentchnick's theory we may suppose that an exceptional will to power has taken hold of a little orphan, and is going to lead him to the formulation of an authoritative philosophical doctrine. In other cases it has led to the exercise of extraordinary political power. If we follow Dr Haynal we may imagine that an exceptionally precocious perception of the fragility of life troubled the mind of the young Descartes over a long period, eventually prompting him to seek a Method for the acquisition of 'sure and certain knowledge'. But a long time had to elapse before that eventuality, and it demanded great perseverance – much more than was required of my farmer as he waited for the harvest.

It was an over-simplification to make a complete distinction between the willed and fruitful loneliness, and unexpected and tragic loneliness, since the latter can also have richly fruitful consequences. Once more we see that the essential thing is not the event – loneliness – but a person's attitude in face of the event. Even in the case of Jesus, when he sought to discover the Father's will in that dark hour in Gethsemane, we can see now that he was not seeking to know if the Father willed his death, but praying that he would accept the death that was coming – which is quite a different matter.

We are back again with the problem that I have been discussing at length in these pages: whether God wills suffering. I make no apology for that, since it is an important problem, especially for the doctor. I understand only too well my colleague who tells me that he is revolted at the idea of a God who was capable of killing his own son. I am convinced that God wills not death, but life; not disease, but healing, and that he is with us in our fight as doctors against death and disease. He has called us simply because in this fallen world there is disease, suffering, and death, and because the important thing is the way men and women face up to this brutal reality.

Jesus himself faced it squarely in all those who were weak, crushed, despised. His Beatitudes are all in the future. The least who will be greatest in the Kingdom of God is in the future. He speaks today as if after the event. I have lived all my working life in this paradoxical perspective of the gospel. So when I was inviting my colleagues just now to look beyond the technical problems in which they are immersed, I ought to have said: look far beyond. That will protect them from impatience and discouragement. For this reason I have made a practice of following the welfare of many of my patients over several decades, and I still do so at the age of eighty-three. I have learned more that way than by treating a larger number of patients for short periods.

I have been well rewarded. I have just been reading the autobiography of one of my patients. Our paths have not crossed these twenty-five years, but as I read her story I marvel at such a wealth of experiences in a single life! From another I receive a moving letter. She has not been spared her meed of suffering. She has had it hard. In psychology, as in dentistry, the treatment hurts as much as the condition it is intended to cure. But today she writes: 'All suffering can bear good fruit.' After the event is sometimes a long time after.

But the nature of fidelity is that it is freely given, and that it does not count on either reward or success. I am happy to pay homage here to the tremendous devotion of the vast majority of my colleagues. Who is the psychoanalyst, however doctrinaire he may be, and whatever his pretensions to being a pure scientist, who, alongside really successful cures, does not persevere with patients with whom he makes scarcely any progress at all? The term 'support psychotherapy' is used with a certain pejorative flavour which is a relic of the contempt in which those suffering from nervous diseases used to be held.

And not only psychoanalysts. I remember a patient, a foreign lady, who used to come and see me occasionally. She told me of the tremendous support her doctor gave her. 'Do you see him often?' I asked. 'Almost every day. He manages to fit me in between two of his patients, or at the end of his surgery. And I often ring him up as well,' she added. 'How long have you been seeing him?' I enquired. She replied, 'Oh, for years!' And who do you think that doctor was? – The professor of medical law at the local university! There are also the 'regulars' who make a practice of ringing the telephone helpline or the Samaritans. They have to be answered and faithfully listened to.

And all the GPs. And the surgeons who deal with the seriously infirm. Despite the fact that they are usually men of action, these surgeons, dedicated to effective intervention, it is wonderful to see the tender solicitude they are capable of. Every doctor feels that to give up a patient because he can do no more for him is to betray his vocation. Such is the power of this 'saviour archetype', which Alphonse Maeder claimed was present in the unconscious of every practitioner.

This is especially true of a country such as Switzerland, which has had the wisdom to safeguard the professional character of medicine. Demagogues claim that the chief object has been to line the doctors' pockets; but that is not true. If a poll were taken, people would be quite surprised at the percentage of free consultations given in this country. Such a poll, however, would not be practicable – no doctor would agree to take part. In any case he would forget some, such as the advice given to the bather who takes the opportunity of approaching him on the beach. The whole pride and joy of all my colleagues is to find people they can help. Even in countries where the bureaucrats try to turn medicine into a great impersonal administrative machine, in their hearts doctors still fight against being turned into state officials.

4

Deprivation and Frustration

When I visited Dr Haynal I told him at the outset that his essay on deprivation had struck me all the more forcibly because the people among whom I work have the vague idea that the aim of psychoanalysis is a life freed from frustration. This may have been true in the beginning when Freud proposed his 'pleasure principle' as the sole motive power of the psychic apparatus. When one really started listening to one life-story after another, one discovered how often psychological disturbances were rooted in an unsatisfied emotional need or an overpowering but unfulfilled desire. There had even been a new theory of education built on it, without rewards or punishments. It was not long, however, before there was a return to the view that a child who meets no resistance is unprepared for the struggle of life. Nevertheless, the idea that frustration is the cause of all our ills has not altogether disappeared.

We know that Freud himself changed his views. From the time of the publication of *Beyond the Pleasure Principle* onwards, he recognized a second principle, that of reality – the reality which stands in the way of our inexhaustible desires; in short, the reality of suffering. All psychoanalysts consider utopian the notion of the 'automatic satisfaction of needs', as Dr Haynal says. We can say we lack a thing without meaning any more than the objective observation that we have not got it, without any emotional connotation. On the other hand the term 'frustration', much used by the psychoanalysts, contains a suggestion of the troubles that can result from it. Seeking a term that would not exclude the idea of the benefits that may flow from the experience, I follow Dr Haynal in using the word deprivation. Another word beloved of the Freudians is 'castration'; but when one reads Françoise Dolto's list in her study of the case of the adolescent Dominique, one realizes that all are varying forms of deprivation.

I ought to put the matter differently: If you recall the distinction I have made between suffering itself and the reaction of the sufferer to his suffering, I shall use the term 'frustration' to denote a destructive reaction, and 'deprivation' to denote the possibility of a creative reaction. You must not suppose that I reject entirely the proposition that the circumstances in which the sufferer finds himself play a part. I am well aware that a destructive reaction is often the only one possible, especially in early childhood, where the helplessness of the infant puts him at the mercy of his parents. Nevertheless we do see quite small children hold out victoriously against them. Sometimes they pay for it with their lives. They use the only weapon they have – crying and screaming. Parents who batter or kill their babies always make the excuse that they could not get them to stop crying.

So we always come back to the dilemma of the two reactions. A whole complex network of innumerable factors, conscious and unconscious, physical, moral, and cultural, determines our behaviour, whether it be destructive or creative. What did surprise me as I read Dr Haynal's essay was the realization that Freud himself had covered much the same ground. Haynal quotes from Freud this profound remark: 'We can lose nothing without replacing it.' With what do we replace it? That is the question. With destructive rebellion, or with creativity?

This second way, however, is not an easy one to take. It requires courage, it requires a whole process of inner maturation which Freud called the work of mourning. Writing about the death of his father, Freud called it 'the most poignant drama of a man's life'. In order not to misunderstand Freud, we must set this remark against what he said about the unconscious desire to kill one's father. We also learn that his favourite reading was Milton's *Paradise Lost*.

There is more to be said, however. There is the Freudian notion of sublimation, about which one may well regret that he did not write more fully. He was cautious. On the subject of creativity, for instance, he writes modestly: 'The essence of the artistic function also remains psychoanalytically inaccessible to us.' Does not the very idea of sublimation express very precisely all that I am talking about in this book? It is the idea of a particular psychic force which has come up against a painful reality, to rebound with equal force in a new direction, like a billiard-ball. The cushion off which the ball has cannoned is deprivation.

Freud, then, seems to be saying that a certain restraint is the source of all creativity and all culture. Philippe Mottu mentions two writers, Pitirim Sorokine, Professor of Sociology at Harvard, and J. D. Unwin, who sought to verify this theory in social history. They were able to show that periods of sexual liberty were the poorest from the cultural point of view, whereas those periods when morality and social convention imposed restrictions on sexual activity were the richest in creative output. This runs counter to what is claimed by the advocates of sexual licence, which is sometimes attributed to the influence of Freud. It is an important lesson for all those who suffer from deprivation of sex life, a deprivation that is exacerbated by these very theories, so that even Roman Catholic priests get married, and burden themselves with psychological problems. For Freud, sublimation is bound up with a deprivation accepted.

What then is this work of mourning of which Freud speaks in *Mourning and Melancholy*? The word 'mourning' is used very generally. We speak of 'mourning a lost opportunity'. The term therefore can cover all kinds of deprivation, though of course it is most usually used in connection with the death of a loved one. Which brings me to my present deprivation – not the distant deprivation of my childhood, but the one I have experienced since my wife's death seven years ago.

As soon as I decided to write this book I realized that I should have to come to this moment. People talk of 'widows and orphans'. I am both. I hesitated for a long time! Because what I have to say is that I have indeed felt a renewal of my creative urge since then. I believe this to be what my friends think too, and that I am not mistaken. What I am afraid of is that many of my readers will be shocked, or think that I can hardly have been very fond of my wife, that it casts a slur on her, and that I am taking my bereavement rather lightly. I have often heard such criticisms levelled at widows and widowers who, instead of sinking into gloom, remain active and serene.

The truth is that this is quite the opposite of a denial of the grief. It really is suffering that I am talking about here, and the creativity of which it may be the occasion. The greater the grief, the greater the creative energy to which it gives rise. I am sure that that is true in my own case. I am nearer those who suffer, and I understand them better. Ah! Growing old alone is quite different from growing old together! What I miss most is the rich dialogue that existed between us.

An important point here is that our dialogue took the form mainly of meditation, which we often practised together, so that we could listen to God in silence, and note down our thoughts, whether they came from ourselves, from our subconscious, or from God, and read them to each other afterwards. It is the surest way to mutual discovery in depth. We used to say to each other things that we should never have said without those very special moments together. I have of course been practising this kind of meditation on my own for nearly fifty years. The one does not take the place of the other. In the past I have often skipped my daily meditation, but since my wife's death I have not missed a single day – as if my rendezvous with God were also a rendezvous with her.

If she had lived, no doubt we should have accommodated ourselves to a quieter mode of life in our old age. I think that there is a certain amount of psychological over-compensation in my present activity, and in my writing so many books. All my work, in any case, could be interpreted as a 'work of mourning'. But I find in it a sort of fellowship with Nelly: we did everything together, and in a way we still do. I have a strong sense of her invisible presence. But what lives in my heart is her new, today's presence, much more than the old one. There are widowers who as it were suspend their lives, as if life had stopped at the moment of their bereavement. Their thoughts have turned towards the past, whereas I live in the present and look to the future.

For some, therefore, it is if anything a retrograde and paralysing presence, whereas my wife's presence is living and stimulating. And not only for me: yesterday my home help said something to me which I found very touching. She still comes on Saturday mornings as she has done ever since before Nelly died. Yesterday she said to me, 'Oh, I do like coming to your house; I have the feeling that your wife is still there, and I keep asking myself how she would want me to do things.' Sociologists, like Jean Ziegler for instance, tell us of the important part played in negro cultures by this consciousness of the presence of the dead amidst the living. What a contrast with our Western civilization which hides and represses the thought of death, so that even mourning clothes are proscribed. Since death is the most characteristic human problem, it is we who are under-developed in this respect.

Since my wife's death I have come to realize that I had lived all my life in mourning, waiting for reunion in heaven with my parents. Nelly had felt that this was so, because just before she died she said to me that she would meet them there. So I have lived my whole life in their unseen presence, in the atmosphere of faith, love, and poetry which characterized their own life. Now, with my new bereavement, my link with heaven is made stronger still, and that stimulates, rather than diminishes, my interest in the problems of this world. The human heart does not obey the rules of logic: it is constitutionally contradictory. I can truly say that I have a great grief and that I am a happy man.

Does that mean that I am in fact performing my work of mourning, in Freud's sense? I do not think so. With Freud it is a detachment, a disinvestment, to borrow a term much used by the psychoanalysts. It is, he writes, a matter of 'severing one's attachment to the object that has been abolished'. So that Dr Lagache, one of his most thoroughgoing disciples, was able to write that it was a matter of 'killing the dead person'. You will see that what I have done is the exact opposite.

You will recall that the mechanism of disinvestment and re-investment was the basis of Freud's theory of sublimation: the billiard ball effect. I could have used a different analogy – the sluice-gate in an irrigation canal, which sends the water in a new direction when it closes. Freud's thought is based on a mechanical model. He is very masculine in that. It is men who turn everything into a mechanism, so that our masculine civilization is like a huge impersonal machine which deper-sonalizes even its individual members and turns them into robots. Freud saw only blind impulses, directed by mechanisms which were also blind. He used the term 'psychic apparatus' to designate the human mind. He gave a series of interpretations of it, both topical and economic, but always in mechanistic terms. So that Paul Ricoeur was able to write: 'The quasi-physical interpretation of the psychic apparatus has never been entirely eliminated from Freudianism.'

It must be remembered that in Freud's day, which was the time of my own childhood, science was at the zenith of its prestige. It has made further immense advances since then, but it has become a lot more modest. Then, it claimed to be the only truth worth putting one's faith in. Virchow had reigned unchallenged over medicine for nearly a century, as Dr Joseph Gander wrote. Then along came Freud, with findings that were radically opposed to the teachings of Virchow. Just imagine – to assert that there were diseases without any anatomico-pathological lesion – it was not scientific!

Freud had therefore to defend himself carefully against the accusation of sinning against science, and of indulging in flights of fancy. Neurotics at that time were after all looked upon as hypochondriacs. In order to get a hearing at all, Freud was compelled rigorously to adopt the rationalist language of science, and he took care to maintain this stance over a long period. There was no sign of purpose in nature, only drives, forces like those of physics, which could be measured so that their mechanisms could be understood. Moreover, this was the cause of the great schism in psychoanalysis, when Jung, his closest collaborator, published his book on the Metamorphoses of the Mind, which was reminiscent of the mode of thought of the alchemists, and when he put forward his theory of the archetypes, which pulled from in front instead of driving from behind.

With Freud we remain strictly in the domain of the quantita-tive, even though it cannot actually be measured. The notion of investment is borrowed from the economists – no strangers to reckoning up quantities. Freud sees only drives in search of 'objects', from the maternal breast to the sex partner and even art, philosophy, and religion. He speaks the language of science, which describes only mechanisms, which tells us what happens but never why it happens. Science presents us with an altogether mechanical picture of the world, like a roundabout which turns ceaselessly but goes nowhere. Everything turns, from the heavenly bodies to the particles of the atomic nucleus, and the endless cycle of cells organizing themselves into living beings and then breaking down in putrefaction. There is a continual receiving of life, transmission of life and movement, and loss of life, with no discernible meaning in it.

I am not criticizing either Freud's scientific work, or science itself, for science by (quite arbitrary) definition excludes considerations of value. A working hypothesis, legitimate as such, which has proved extremely useful. But one comes in the end to what has been predicated to start with – the absence of any meaning in the interminable round of phenomena, because meaning belongs to the order of values. Jacques Monod is reduced to invoking *Chance and Necessity*, and that is a pure act of faith. Most scientists now recognize the limitations of science: that it explains mechanisms, but not the mystery of the world and of the human person. Science is an effective handmaid of medicine, but medicine is not only science.

In any case, Freud was too much of a doctor not to ask himself in the evening of his life questions quite foreign to the rigorous parameters of science. He had won his battle. Psychoanalysis had been integrated into medicine. He was able to give free rein to his thought. He did not put forward as scientific theory his hypothesis of a primitive murder in *Totem and Taboo*, nor his studies on 'the future of an illusion', on Moses and monotheism, or on the myth of Eros and Thanatos. Several of his followers reproached him for it. Though I do not share his views in the matter, I think it is altogether to his honour that he did not allow himself to be boxed in.

But we can at least enter into dialogue. Thus, it seems to me that what Freud missed in this perspective of investment and disinvestment is the difference between material investment, which can be measured, and spiritual investment, which cannot. If I have a penny, and I give it away, I no longer have it. We all learn that in early life, when a brother or sister takes some toy of ours, and we protest: 'No! It's mine!' But if I have love, and I give it to someone else, I have more as a result. If I have courage and I give it to one of my patients, I end up with more courage. If I have faith and impart it to another, my own faith is increased. That seems to me to mark the irreducible distance between the material and the spiritual worlds.

What I think Freud missed is the spiritual dynamic, which is different from the dynamics of physics – at any rate within the limitations which have up to now been imposed on that science, if I am to believe the physicists Jean E. Charon and his book *L'esprit, cet inconnu*, which I read with enormous interest. Indeed, I have just been evoking this contrast between material and spiritual economy by my analogies and in my usual manner of speaking. But, with Charon, I could have said it in the language of physics: material economy tends always towards the increase of entropy in accordance with the second law of thermodynamics; whereas the economy of the spirit tends always to the increase of order. The electron, the particle which 'forms a veritable universe in itself', is the 'bearer of the spirit', and is characterized by 'a space which is increasingly distinct from our material space in which the process of evolution involves a continual degradation of information and order'.

The two economies, according to Charon, can thus be expressed mathematically, in inverse formulae. The material economy is exhaustible, while the spiritual economy can be enriched – which is as much as to say, it seems to me, that the former leads towards the end of the world, and the latter towards immortality. Pastor Henry Babel has attempted a most interesting comparison between the physical concepts of entropy and order, and the teachings of the great religions. The present energy crisis and the reports of the Club of Rome clearly illustrate the contrast. We are witnessing the failure of a civilization which has relied only on material values. In a lecture on the subject of Moses, Dr Richardeau explains this in psychoanalytical terms: the consumer society belongs to Freud's 'oral stage'; we cling to it like the baby to his mother's breast, for the satisfaction of our most primitive needs.

Jesus warned us that the treasures of this earth are subject to corruption and theft, unlike those of heaven (Matt. 6.19). The more energy I expend, the less I have; the more moral energy I expend, the more I have. Who does not see that love is expandable, but not measurable? How then can we talk of a need to disinvest love in order to be able to reinvest it?

What of St Francis of Assisi, St Vincent de Paul, and Mother Teresa in our own day? Do you think they had to disinvest? On the contrary, the more open the heart is to love, the more its love increases. What about all the doctors, including Freud himself, and you – psychoanalysts, and all the others who devote their lives to the service of those who suffer! That is why I have not needed to follow the advice of Dr Lagache, of whom I was talking just now, and why the lively love that I still have for my wife, so far from shutting me in, gives me new energy to follow my vocation. In any case Dr Lagache would have refrained from giving me his advice, because of my age.

Indeed, I do not offer myself as an example to younger men. It is obvious that a widower in the prime of life who is thinking of remarrying must 'sever his attachment to the object that has been abolished', as Freud said – although I am not happy with this use of the word 'object' instead of 'person'. It is a shocking fate for a second wife to feel that her husband is still attached to the first, or even that he is pretending to be so out of a quite misplaced sense of loyalty. It is equally cruel for him to refuse the second wife a child. I am the issue of the second marriage of my father. It would be wrong of me not to point that out.

I think that as we grow old we are called upon to open our hearts more widely, in every circumstance to move on from the rather self-centred love of youth to a more disinterested love. This double aspect – self-centred and altruistic – although an apparent contradiction, is a feature of all love. Love is a spontaneous movement, it does not weigh up pros and cons, it will even sacrifice itself for the beloved person or cause. But it is also selfish, in that it seeks the satisfaction of an instinct – the sex instinct, or the maternal, paternal, or social instincts. When you come to think of it, we should not care to be loved in a totally disinterested fashion, so that the person who loved us took no pleasure in doing so.

It is the respective proportions of these two tendencies in love that can alter. In youth, with our lives in front of us and a natural aspiration to make a success of them, we love those who are useful to us, those who encourage and love us. A child at school will love maths if he gets good marks in it. He will take pleasure in working at it, and so get even better marks. He is fond of the teacher, and for his part the teacher likes the pupil whose progress and admiration he finds flattering. Such interlocking systems of reciprocal love are a feature of the whole of our working lives. Even the hardest work can seem light if we love the people for whom we are working, whether employers, customers, or partners. The same work can feel like a ball and chain if the opposite is the case. But when we have retired, when we have left behind the lists of competition, we can enlarge the horizons of our love.

Love that is self-interested rapidly degenerates into possessiveness; and while unselfish love can do miracles, possessive love can just as readily bring about catastrophes. It is possessiveness which makes a husband forbid his wife to take part in all kinds of activities in which she would like to find fulfilment. It is possessive love which makes a mother watch over her child like a broody hen, and prevent him from becoming adult. The thing that strikes me is that such mothers are quite unaware of the harm that their possessiveness does to a child, often a favourite child, so convinced are they that it is for the child's own good that they watch over him and shield him from every risk.

At the same time, because of its exclusiveness sexual love is normally possessive, and this gives it something in common with the material economy I was talking about just now; because it has a physical side, the giving of the body, so that the psychoanalytical notion of investment is justified in this respect. That this physical commitment is exclusive, is not only a law imposed by traditional morality or by society; it is inscribed in the human heart. The most inconstant man swears eternal love to his latest conquest. And he means it! To choose one woman is to renounce all the others as sexual partners; not, of course, the desire which is part of his nature, but its unfettered satisfaction. All men desire all women – which many women find it hard to understand.

Unlike a woman, a man often claims, in order to justify his conduct, that he can easily love two women at the same time. He may even tell his wife, if she discovers his sceret, that it is in her interest to shut her eyes to it, because it makes him nicer to her. But loving is more than being nice. And in the atmosphere of frankness that belongs to the doctor's consulting-room he is willing to admit that it is not the same love. In order to forestall misunderstanding, I add that though Jesus said that no man must put asunder what God had joined together (Matt. 19.6), he was just as severe, if not more so, about those who judge others (Luke 6.37). And I remind you that to both those who condemn and those who are condemned, he brings the good news of God's grace.

There is, then, a certain contrast between sexual love, bound up with our instincts, and love pure and simple, which answers to the call of the spirit. The first is exclusive and implies an exclusive investment of the libido. The second is quite the opposite – it belongs to the economy of the spirit, which is radically anti-exclusive and tends towards the extension of the area of love. If you think that it too is a matter of instinct, I invite you to read the work of a geneticist such as Richard Dawkins, who shows in his book *The Selfish Gene* that we are programmed for selfishness by our genetic code. If that is a truth which surprises the idealist, I do not think it will surprise doctors, whose vocation turns them into realists.

5

The Difficulties and Delays of Acceptance

The Bible too is realistic. It has no illusions about man's selfishness. Nevertheless it asserts that with his own breath God has communicated to selfish man an aspiration towards disinterested love. Hence the permanent conflict in which we are all engaged between our genetic code and the need for a supernatural love which we have received from God. For Christians, the solution is in the fresh outpouring of the Spirit, sent by Jesus. St Paul says that love is one of the fruits of the spirit (Gal. 5.22), and St John that it comes from God: 'everyone who loves is begotten by God' (I John 4.7). They are echoing Jesus and his command, 'Love one another' (John 13.34).

Moreover, all the great religions are at one in teaching love. I wondered, for instance, whether it was not precisely because the Buddha was a sensitive child, deeply hurt by his mother's death – and thus imbued with a precocious understanding of the fragility of our human condition – that his father had shut him up in his palace in order to shield him from all encounter with sickness, poverty, old age, and death. And there it was – it was precisely this encounter which made him into the Buddha, the enlightened one, who had long meditated upon this problem of suffering which concerns us, and had found that the only answer is in disinterested love, in renunciation, in the willing acceptance of deprivation. For the truth is that the problem of deprivation is not to be solved by shutting one's eyes, but by facing it courageously.

Erich Fromm, in his book *The Art of Loving*, also asserts, from the psychological point of view, the primacy of brotherly love – susceptible of universal extension, and disinterested, as it is – over sexual love, which inevitably retains the self-seeking character of an instinct in pursuit of its own satisfaction. This is not in any sense to imply condemnation of sex. Eric Fuchs has pointed out that this attitude of condemnation which has been such a dead weight upon the church for so long, and which it has at last begun to throw off, was due to the influence of stoicism, which was at its height during the first few centuries of Christianity, Christianity triumphed, but there took place a phenomenon pointed out by Jung – the victor always inherits the demon of the vanquished.

Obviously sex is creative in procreation, as the word itself indicates. But it is also creative as a factor in the formation of the person: often it constitutes the first initiation into the making of a personal relationship, into the triumph of brotherly love over the radical selfishness programmed by the genetic code, and then leads to the spiritual experience *par excellence* which is the encounter with God, the altogether Other.

Laurence and Jacques de Bourbon Busset bear witness to this, interviewed by Christian Chabanis on the existence of God: 'When we met,' says the husband, 'we were both agnostics, but our mutual attachment opened out new perspectives for us . . . Strictly human love has opened new horizons for us. We discovered – that is what happened in my case – that there was more to life than calculation, rationality, argument: that there existed a world of self-giving.' His wife adds: 'I came to

God via the idea of eternal life, immediately I said to myself: it is not possible that a reality which I feel to be so strong, so indestructible, should cease to exist because of the distintegration of a few cells.' And a little further on: 'It is through our love for each other that we can share in God ... wherever people love each other, some may not realize it, but they share in God, even without knowing it.'

Unfortunately this development of conjugal love into the experience of the love of God does not always happen, as Bovet pointed out in his book on marriage. There are many couples, some married, some not, whose life together is no more than the association of two egoists. Their sex life may be successful and satisfying to the sexual love of both, but they have never enjoyed the spiritual experience of real personal contact. They may tell us triumphantly, even in the midst of marital conflict: 'Oh, our sex life, *that*'s all right!' The fact is that it is not all right: it may be providing the satisfaction of an instinct, but it has left unfulfilled its function in the development of the person. It has in fact remained only a mechanism. It is possible to have technical success and existential failure – and sex will not stave off marital disaster. At the same time, the existential function of sex can be realized through social contact between the sexes, and brotherly friendship.

What is the spiritual? It is what goes beyond all mechanisms and the limitations of their selfish investment. It is communion. For me it means a personal relationship with God through intimacy with Jesus Christ. But it is always the triumph of love over one's 'high horse', as a friend of mine used to say; it is always the casting away of the mask behind which we protect our real selves.

It is also communion with our fellows, with nature, and with beauty, with all that belongs to that non-material, non-mechanical economy of which I was talking, and which defies the limitations of investment. Do you think a painter ought to distance himself from his early works in order to invest his talent in a search for something new? In every studio there is an old canvas which the artist has refused to sell, and from which he draws creative inspiration in his love of beauty. My own first book has aged considerably over the last forty years. I could not write it now as I wrote it then, and I am quite embarrassed when a student questions me on the subject of typology – I abandoned my researches into it a long time ago. But I have never wanted to revise the book. It is like a cry from my youth, burning with the experiences I had had. Can one understand an author without reading his first book?

It is also communion with suffering which has no limits, and the personal courage to accept suffering and deprivation. I was thinking about that yesterday evening, dining alone at my little table, the only one to be alone in the spacious dining-room of a hotel in Palma. And the only one among all these holiday-makers to be at work, as I am every day on this book. Many women on their own have told me that they have given up such holidays because they could not bear dining alone like that among all the starry-eyed couples and the noisy parties. I have heard some widowers say the same.

I observe all these tourists. I know that they all have their problems, often tragic ones. Many more problems than most of you think, because you are not as well placed as I am to know life as it is. And also because everyone hides his problems for lack of someone on whom to unload them. These holiday-makers have provisionally laid their problems aside, aided by the distractions of holidays and collective stimulus. And each one plays his little game in an effort at least to look happy, if not actually to be so. There is even more to it: sometimes in order to be happy it is necessary to seem the opposite, in order to attract sympathy.

Then I reflected that I was surely one of the happiest of us all; because I was in a state of creativity. Who will deny that in order to be so one has also to be in tune with oneself, to accept one's lot and one's deprivations? Happy also because I hope that some lonely person, reading my book, will take heart, pluck up courage, and become more creative once more instead of withdrawing into deeper gloom. Probably not to write a book! And yet, why not? You can start at any age, as with painting, or chess. Everyone to his taste. Simply, perhaps, a little more creative of himself, of his own person, evolving towards serenity, towards accepting his life as it is, transforming a loneliness suffered passively and with bitterness into a solitude that is welcomed and made to bear fruit.

Then I wrote all this down during my meditation this morning, along with other more intimate items, of course. If you are, philosophically, a Cartesian, you will be asking me whether it really came from God. I do not claim that, but I reckon that the main thing is that one approaches him, at the same time noting one's thoughts with a certain critical reserve, but not too much, seeking the truth, for all truth comes from God.

It is scarcely easier to accept the truth about ourselves and also our limitations in the search for it, than to accept our deprivations. In the end of the day, to do the work of mourning, for Freud as well as for me, is to accept reality. This was the turning-point in Freud's work, when to the pleasure principle he added the principle of reality. In the realm of experience, then, Freud and I are at one. Theories and doctrines divide men. Feelings unite them. Happiness often does so, and so does suffering, which no one escapes. Freud suffered terribly in the course of his last illness and all his operations. 'I cannot stand any more!' he murmured. How near to him that makes me feel!

Near to him, and to all those who suffer, with whom I have been in contact throughout my career, with whom I have sympathized, and who have taught me practically everything I know about life by allowing me to share their suffering. Near also to some unknown reader who is going to read what I am writing, and who is suffering undeservedly from some deprivation – from sickness, disability, remorse, or some cruel grief. And see how delicate a problem it is: I only have to tell him that we have to accept, and he is hurt! At once he would feel that he is cut off from me, that I do not understand him; he would have the impression that I do not know how much he is suffering. 'We must accept' is easy to say when you are not suffering, or not suffering as much. I do not think I have ever said it to anyone.

And yet at this point in our meditation on the trials of life, I have to say something about accepting them. Acceptance plays such an important part in our development that I come back to it in every book I write. It was already the main theme in my first, *The Healing of Persons*. As soon as I asked myself which diseases pertained to the whole person rather than just to a bodily lesion or to some disturbed psychological function, the thing that struck me was the harmful effect of any kind of rejection: non-acceptance of one's age, one's sex, a spouse or a parent, an affliction, a failure, a mistake one had made – in short, rejection of one's lot in life. So I spoke of acceptance; but in my youthful zeal I tended to treat it as black and white; I failed to see that there were shades in between, and that a long apprenticeship was necessary. As I have just said, to preach acceptance to someone in revolt is to aggravate his distress.

The first point to notice is that acceptance is much more difficult for some people than for others. They are usually people disposed to self-doubt by the circumstances of their childhood. They are lacking in self-confidence and in the sense of security that every person needs, so that any difficult event causes them to go to pieces. There are even some, as I have often observed, who put up with serious troubles quite well, but find the little contrarieties of social life very hard to bear. The most trivial slight seriously upsets them. My wife was like that. Then she blamed herself for finding it harder than I did to accept such things, in which she was quite unfair to herself since there was no merit in it on my part; but it set up a vicious circle and made acceptance even harder for her.

So, though no one said to her, 'You must accept,' she said it to herself and blamed herself for not succeeding. What is wrong with the saying, which has sometimes been attributed to me, is the 'must', turning as it does acceptance into an order, a moral law, or even a simple friendly piece of advice. One does not accept to order; acceptance never comes from outside, through giving in to prompting by someone else, but from inside, from a slow inner evolution.

Further, it is obvious that some of the knocks that life brings us are harder than others, and consequently more difficult to accept. We lack objectivity when we talk abstractly about the trials of life as if they were all comparable. I was seventy-six when I lost my wife. It is quite a different thing to lose a wife at the age of forty. There are similar differences in the death of a child, depending on the age of the child. But the biggest distinction to be made is according to whether the misfortune which befalls us comes from natural causes or from the injustice of our fellow men. In the latter case acceptance may be culpable weakness, which obviously raises a serious crisis of conscience of the sort which I described in my book *To Resist or to Surrender?*, but which only the person concerned can settle. You know the inner struggle that Jesus himself had to go through in Gethsemane (Matt. 26.36).

There are acceptances that only God can demand of us, because it is also his love which makes acceptance possible and leads us towards it. Then, is the work of mourning the work of God? I am convinced that it is so. Nobody ever told me to accept being an orphan; or my widowhood now – and many other griefs in between. Who, then, helped me? I told you just now: those who loved me enough to reveal to me the love of God. One does not help people to accept the trials of life by preaching at them, but by loving them.

That is a universal truth: believers do not have a monopoly of love. It is not so much a matter of telling our patients of the love of God, as of loving them ourselves. Jesus made that quite clear. Think of that simple parable of his in which he tells of a father who asks his two sons to go and work in his vineyard. One says yes, but does not go; the other says no, but goes (Matt. 21.28). Like the second of these is the doctor who calls himself an unbeliever, but has so much love for his patients that without knowing it he is for them the revealer of God's love.

But acceptance also requires a delay which one must not fail to recognize. That is why I felt that Monique Kressmann's intervention, of which I was telling you just now, was so important. Thoughts can go beyond time, whereas the feelings are enslaved by it. By means of thought we can see the belated fruits of affliction, or the creativity that may flow from deprivation. I am writing this book very largely for my colleagues and for all those who, like them, come to the aid of the afflicted; in order to invite them to take a longer view, to see the harvest of the future, and so to be encouraged in the work they have to do today.

But we have not yet reached that harvest; we are only in the time of ploughing. To talk of acceptance at the time of suffering and revolt is to put up a barrier between ourselves and our patients, because that distant vision is still impossible for them. We must walk in step with them. This is the time for sympathy and understanding of our patients' anger. Fortunately it is quite possible fully to live this moment with our patients while at the same time looking further ahead, and that is perhaps the key to psychotherapy, as it is of teaching. There is a lot of ground to cover before we reach the goal of genuine acceptance. I have seen people force themselves into premature acceptance, even persuade themselves that they have accepted when in reality they are only repressing their anger under pressure from some other person or even from themselves.

Let us look, for instance, at the supreme acceptance – that of death. Elisabeth Kubler-Ross has thrown a flood of light on the subject. She has devoted herself to talking to sick people who are near to death, so as to give them an opportunity of talking about their feelings and about what is on their minds. Up to now, doctors, relatives, and friends have always tried to keep off the subject, in the belief that it is necessary to distract the patient in order to maintain his morale. In fact, as Madame Kubler-Ross has shown, it is we who have been afraid of real dialogue at such times, and of the emotions it arouses. She even mentions the pastor who reads a psalm because that is easier to do than to enter into personal dialogue. That reminds me of a remark by Michael Balint concerning some of our medical actions: Whom are you trying to reassure, he asks, your patient or yourself? In fact I can remember dying people to whom I have listened with enough attention for them to have the courage to open their hearts to me, and for me to make a sincere response. They are not numerous, but I shall never forget them.

Madame Kubler-Ross describes the stages in this evolution towards death. At first there is the shock when the patient learns or guesses that there is no hope of recovery. Next he goes through a stage of refusal: he is unwilling to believe it. Then comes rebellion and anger: Why me? Why now? But the anger is impotent, and he moves into discouragement and depression. Then comes a new phase, which the author calls the bargaining stage, as if the patient hoped to placate fate by means of submission and renunciation. It is after this long pilgrimage that Madame Kubler-Ross sees the sick person arrive at peaceful acceptance. There often takes place at that point a change which she calls decathexis, a sort of distancing, as if the dying person already did not altogether belong in the world of the living. Then there is no further need to speak, only affectionately to hold the dying person's hand.

As you see, all liberating growth takes time. With variations, we can see Madame Kubler-Ross's stages in the approach to every reality which is hard to accept. We doctors see it in the majority of our patients. They start with a phase of refusal; they do not want to recognize that they are ill, and often make incredible efforts to continue their normal lives as if they were in good health. I have done so myself on occasion. Sometimes their families have to use all sorts of subterfuges to get them to come and see us. Then come anger and revolt. Oh, yes! It is very important for them to be able to express these feelings and for them to feel that we understand. There is no question yet of acceptance.

Or there is the young woman who has undergone the shock of a broken engagement, and who knows that at her age she will have little chance of marriage. She heroically denies her grief, and assures me that she can live happily without husband or children. She is sincere, and I can congratulate her, for I know that happiness depends more on ourselves than on the circumstances of our lives. But she has by no means yet reached the stage of real acceptance of the fact that she will remain single, and I shall for several years still see her going through periods of anger, of depression, and 'bargaining', before she achieves acceptance.

Didier Duruz, a research student at the Institut d'Etudes Sociales, wrote a report in which he adapted Madame Kubler-Ross's model for the acceptance of old age. It is a theme on which I am very frequently asked to speak, since in my country the big corporations, both private and public, organize seminars for their personnel on the subject of preparation for retirement. I find this work particularly interesting, since it gives me an opportunity of meeting a quite different audience from the ones I am accustomed to addressing in universities, parishes, and societies, which represent only a tiny section of the community. The rest hardly ever come to hear such talks, thinking that they are only meant for intellectuals; but when they do they are surprised to find that they deal with problems that are common to all, such as what is the purpose of life when all at once retirement brings to an end the work that has given meaning to one's existence for so many years.

The sudden realization of the inexorable advance of old age also comes with a shock. I remember very well the first time that a charming young lady got up to offer me her seat in a bus! Ah! I was no longer in her eyes a man from whom she might expect a complimentary gesture of politeness, but an old man to whom she was offering a gesture of charity.

However, the shock of which Didier Duruz writes in his research paper is not only that which is experienced by an ageing man such as I was then. It is also the shock which he himself received when as a young social welfare student he did a course in geriatry, and suddenly found himself confronted with a picture of old age which society prefers to hide from public view – the sight of a group of twenty old people in complete physical, and especially mental, decline. My immediate thought was that his research project had been a kind of therapeutic enterprise, undertaken in order to cure himself of the effects of that shock. At the *viva*, when he had to defend his thesis, I was a member of the examining board, and I likened his experience to that of the Buddha, whose father's solicitude had shielded him for a long time from such spectacles, rather after the fashion in which our Western society shuts up the sick, the infirm, the poor, and the old away from everyday life.

Thus in Duruz's paper one is reading two stories at once – one is the account of the old people he is observing and who may gradually reach acceptance through all the stages described by Madame Kubler-Ross, and the other is the story of Didier Duruz himself, who through nine months of study (is not the figure the very symbol of creativity?) gradually came to an understanding of the meaning of life: passing from 'having' to 'being', from the avidity of youth and middle age through all kinds of renunciations – deprivations – to seeking one's identity in oneself and not in what one does, acquires, or possesses. 'One must look upon growing old,' he writes, 'as a sort of forced passage towards being, towards being fully born,' This last expression he borrows from Erich Fromm.

For of course not all the old people Duruz met were lamentable wrecks. He met others, hidden away just the same, who impressed him quite as much, because they radiated life and peace, happiness even, despite their infirmity and their lack of everything that our contemporaries are so proud of – knowledge, wealth, prestige, energy, and power. I am reminded of one of my first patients, at a time when I was still a houseman at the Policlinic, working as a Social Security doctor. She was an aged English spinster who had somehow – I never found out how – ended up paralysed in her chair in a miserable room in the slums of Geneva. Her only visitors were the district nurse, Mlle Wehrlin, and myself. But it was always a joy to see her. I always came away with my store of courage and joy replenished. It was very clear that her secret lay in her acceptance, and that the source of that acceptance was in her faith. That fascinated me, because my own faith then was more theoretical than living.

6

Anger

So, all these misfortunes of which I write are not only the ones
which we personally experience, but also those which befall
others and which move us as much as our own. Our patients
are magic mirrors in which we see our own human condition.
There are some patients whom I cannot treat without saying
to myself, 'I hope to goodness nothing like this happens to
me!' Or if it is an old person, 'I hope I don't finish up like this!'
At my age I am well aware that it is not so much death we are
afraid of, as the manner in which it may come – the pain, and
most of all the decline into senility. Is that a special kind of conceit? I suppose it is, and I can see that I ought also to accept
that my death may not come in the way that I should have
preferred.

But there are also people like my old English spinster, who
make one think, 'I only hope I shall be able to stay as serene as
that, with her acceptance and her faith!' Conceit again? Yes, of
course. Ecclesiastes would call it vanity (Eccl. 1.2). There is
more to it, however: the intuitive perception of a law of life.
Rebellion is contagious, but so is acceptance. Blessed is he who
can accept: for himself, first, because he finds inner peace; but
for others as well, because he helps them to accept.

Nevertheless there is no contradiction between anger and
acceptance, as it might seem to our too logical minds. Logic
has nothing to do with feelings. Anger and acceptance are

contradictory in theory, but in practice they hold hands like the dancers in a folk-dance. Madame Kubler-Ross, Didier Duruz, and all the psychoanalysts teach us that one does not reach acceptance except through rebellious anger, beyond the anger and after giving vent to it. The greatest obstacle to acceptance is anger that has been repressed because one has not dared to give expression to it. Psychotherapy frequently only becomes truly liberating after the explosion of anger that has been bottled up. Dr Arthur Janov has made it the basis of his technique by allowing it to be expressed not only in words but also in dramatic gestures.

I am reminded of a conference session on the medicine of the person in which a young colleague who was talking about his unhappy childhood suddenly gave vent to such a brutal burst of anger against his mother that the whole audience felt acutely embarrassed. I was in the chair, and could see the surreptitious glances that many of my friends were throwing in my direction, as if pleading with me: 'Stop him, it's almost unbearable!' But I remained silent, knowing that people do not come to such meetings as they do to ordinary medical conferences, to listen to polished scientific expositions – very useful, of course, but stripped of all personal emotion. On the contrary, I know that they come to be initiated into the secret of personal contact, and that for that to happen one must enter into it oneself, and overcome one's own fear of emotion.

Didier Duruz has a lot to say about anger. He tells a striking story: he goes to see a poor old man whose decent, ordinary, happy life has been shattered by a series of cruel blows – the divorce of his daughter, his own enforced retirement, his wife's death, and a stroke which has left him unable to speak. Real conversation is impossible, especially since he is of Italian extraction, and the few words that come back to him halt between French and Italian. His loneliness is complete; he no longer frequents his usual café, because nobody understands what he is trying to say. How can contact be re-established when dialogue is impossible? Carried away by the strength of his emotion, Duruz mutters over and over again, 'It's not fair! It's not fair!', banging on the table with his fist to emphasize each word. And he sees the old man's eyes light up. He has been able to join him in his anger.

Anger must be expressed. The thought struck me forcibly during Didier Duruz's *viva* – all those professors, students and social workers constantly confronted by the injustices and the red tape of modern life, the way they made common cause in their anger, returning to the subject constantly, because Duruz had had the courage to talk about his own anger; anger against the 'principle of reification which is so deeply ingrained in our society', even against the 'medical establishment which rules unquestioned inside our institutions', and against many more such things.

I have just been reading an exciting book: *Mars*, by Fritz Zorn – a pseudonym which means 'Fritz Anger'. His anger is the very same as that of the social workers I have just mentioned, except that he is the son of a rich Zürich family from the 'Rive Dorée', the fashionable quarter of the city. What an indictment of the all-powerful conformist, conventional mentality in my country – it can stifle any chance of personal life, of becoming a person, just as surely up there at the top of the social scale as down among the outcasts dealt with by the social services.

Fritz Anger has written his book at the age of thirty-two, when he is actually dying of cancer, or more precisely, of a malign lymphoma. He even thinks that this organic disease is the 'natural' outcome of the disease from which he has suffered since childhood, and which he calls, for want of another name, 'depression'. That, of course, he puts forward only as a personal idea of his own. One cannot argue the point, because nothing is known of the cause of cancer, beyond the fact that there is a range of circumstances in which it may arise. I recall my astonishment at the visit of an American colleague who thought that the cause of cancer was psychological.

However that may be, Fritz Anger is able to write that he is better since he has been ill, that he is relieved to be officially recognized as having a disease that has a name, when for thirty years he has been ill without knowing it, or at least without knowing what his sickness was – an undefined illness which I might well call the disease of not being a person. He describes the circles in which he lived, where everything was sacrificed to the need for harmony. In order to have a harmonious life, without conflicts, both in the family and in relation to those outside, one had to give up having any personal opinions of one's own, so that one became incapable of having any.

When one asked one's mother a question, she replied ambiguously until she knew what her husband's view was, so as not to disagree with him, but even his opinion was not his own personal, considered view, but rather a collective opinion, a collection of prejudices common to all the members of the set in which they moved. It followed that all those subjects which demand a personal judgment – religion, money, sex – were taboo. The excuse was made that these questions were 'too complicated', and were best not argued about. At such a price was harmony preserved, a harmony without any discordant note, an impersonal humming, without any real personal life. The author can truthfully say that he never had any problem with his parents!

A good boy, nicely behaved towards everybody, but incapable of loving. He was able to do well at university, take a doctorate, become a teacher, write plays that made audiences laugh – though he never laughed, though he was bored to death, and was sinking into lonely depression. He had only begun to live a little more of a personal life, with the help of a course of psychotherapy, when he discovered with horror the emptiness that was hidden behind the facade imposed by his surroundings, when he gave vent to the anger repressed into his unconscious, and wrote this masterpiece, just before he died. There's creativity for you!

Open the Bible: Moses, Job, the authors of the psalms, the prophets – there is plenty of righteous anger there. Jesus himself overturning the tables of the money-changers in the Temple. You will accuse me of the mistake of confusing anger against men and their iniquities, and anger against God. Unfortunately the boundary between them is not so precise. Since we can only conceive of God as all-powerful, both we and our patients, believers as well as unbelievers, impute to him in the last analysis everything we cannot accept, catastrophes both natural and social. Though Moses smashes the tablets of the Law before the golden calf (Ex. 32.19), he has fought hard beside the burning bush against God and against the mission to which God was calling him (Ex. 3.11). And the most timid of the prophets, such as Jeremiah, flare up against God when he constrains them to prophesy and to incarnate his own anger. And in the Psalms we find a dramatic mixture of flights of adoration and imprecations against God. Holy Writ is full of conflicts, conflicts between men, and between God and men, and when true harmony – the harmony of faith – supervenes, it is only after an explosion of anger.

You are thinking perhaps too that I am neglecting the necessary light and shade in talking of anger instead of dispute, argument, anxiety, and questioning. My thinking prompts me to take a less sophisticated line – for me, acceptance says 'yes'; all the rest say 'no'. And does not the fundamental ambiguity of human nature derive from the fact that 'yes' and 'no' are inevitably connected? One example which to me seems very telling, is the contrast between the two last words of Jesus on the cross: 'My God, my God, why have you deserted me?' (Matt. 27.46), and 'Father, into your hands I commit my spirit' (Luke 23.46). Right to the end Jesus met this tension between 'no' and 'yes' which is inherent in our human existence. It seems to me that every act of rebellion conceals an unconscious aspiration towards acceptance, and that every act of acceptance is still hot from the rebellion which gave rise to it.

Many people have said to me that they could not believe in God because of the anger they felt in face of the ravages of evil, in face of all the innocent victims of natural disasters and human injustice. I have no answer for them; but they have always appeared to me to be unconscious believers, beginners of course, but believers nevertheless. After interviewing famous scientists on the question of the existence of God, Christian Chabanis puts the question to Marie-Jeanne Pontal, a ninety-year-old widow who has lost her only daughter. He asks her if in her grief she has been tempted to blame God. She answers, 'When we blame him, that means that we still believe he exists.' I too used to feel that some of my patients who claimed to be atheists took God more seriously than some believers. They took seriously what the Bible says and what we repeat – that God is love. That's the beginning of a creed, anyway.

Be that as it may, in the personal history of many believers a holy rebellion has been the first step towards a trusting encounter with God; and we are told that he himself was angry, and relented (Ex. 32.14). One of my own most precious friendships was born out of a dispute. And in practice I have often had occasion to reassure believers who have felt rebellion stirring once again in their hearts against a misfortune that they thought they had finally accepted – a tragic bereavement, for instance, or their failure to marry, or some infirmity. They blame themselves, considering it a setback in their faith. On the contrary, however, it is the sign of greater maturity, a stage on the road to more complete acceptance.

There is, then, a sort of dialectic between 'no' and 'yes'. There are indeed people who can say 'yes' without hesitation in the midst of misfortune, especially children. It is a gift of grace. But very often there is a struggle, and the 'yes' only comes as a hard won victory over 'no'. One senses that at once. There is a marked contrast between such cases, and the person who says with an air of capitulation, 'What's the use? You've got to put up with it.' Then it is no more than resignation: a passive, gloomy, sterile attitude, a sort of admission of failure, or, to put it in psychological terms, of repression. True acceptance, on the other hand, is active, creative, the source of powerful development of the person. That is what gives it its grandeur. It is in this sense that Goethe said that there is no situation that cannot be ennobled either by action or by acceptance.

I have an excellent friend, a medical colleague, who underwent an operation for a very painful condition. Naturally, when I went to visit him he talked about his experience. At the point when he was in greatest pain, he told me, the thought came to him that not only had he to accept his suffering, he had to 'get inside it'. I was struck by the expression. It meant so much more than the rather tame idea of acceptance, which too many people confuse with resignation. His expression evoked a much more vigorous reaction – like a courageous dive off the edge!

'Get inside it'! I have often quoted my friend's remark in seminars on preparation for retirement. A new page is to be turned, and it needs to be turned resolutely. One cannot read two pages at once. The resigned 'got to put up with it' of those who only half-heartedly accept retirement – as well as the old age which it heralds – leaves them passive, divided, and bitter. It is a matter of accepting the challenge of life which always requires a fresh burst of enthusiasm, a vigorous effort at adaptation, a new personal development.

No longer should we look upon retirement as a dimming of the lights, a 'well-earned rest', to use the stupid phrase of well-wishers at retirement parties – for prolonged rest invites inertia, decline, and decay. Sitting in an armchair awaiting visits which do not come is another form of passive and sterile acceptance, a sort of capitulation. As you will see, it is a good illustration of the problem of deprivation which we are studying together in this book. The retired person is suddenly deprived of the occupational activity which for so many years held a preponderant place in his life, and which has stimulated him with its imperious demands. And with it he also loses all the social relationships it involved, as well as the prestige which is conferred upon him by his competence and his responsibilities, or at least the esteem which attaches to all paid work in our profit-conscious civilization. With all these deprivations, the time has come for personal creativity, a time to rediscover the creative imagination which is so exuberant in the child, now stifled by years of routine, of thought, of making plans.

The same applies to all other kinds of deprivation. Right at the start of adult life it is necessary to say goodbye to youth, to devote all one's strength to one's career and to the building of a family home. The same call to creative renewal rings out at every one of the trials that beset us on our way through life, each of which marks an irreversible turning-point. Widowhood, or some similar cruel bereavement; an accident or a serious illness, a failure or a betrayal; life thereafter will never be what it was. It is not enough to resign oneself to the inevitable. The new stage of life must be undertaken and not just undergone. One must know what one wants to do, and above all what one wants to become, oneself. 'Getting inside it' means committing oneself completely, living the present moment. That implies a revision of values, a search for fresh inspiration.

Then the 'work of mourning' takes on a quite different dimension from that which Freud gave it, a spiritual dimension which only the spiritual life can confer upon it. Freud's purely psychological definitions: 'severing one's attachment to the object that has been abolished' seems very passive, very pale, compared with the intensely creative event that is spiritual acceptance, in which 'yes' to suffering merges into 'yes' to God. This is especially true of Christian acceptance; for Jesus' message is realistic and hard. He speaks of the sword and of persecution, and of forsaking all. 'If anyone wants to be a follower of mine, let him renounce himself and take up his cross and follow me' (Matt. 16.24). His words touch us because he accepted the cross himself, and because every trial accepted brings us nearer to him.

I was moved when I came across the expression 'to carry one's cross' from the pen of a Jewish writer, André Chouraqui. He is a pious and fervent Jew, faithful to his religion but respectful of our Christian faith, as well as of the faith of Islam. His prophetic appeal for a rapprochement of our three biblical religions engages my full support. When I spoke in a Teheran mosque at the invitation of Ayatollah Tabatabai, I was able to tell all those Moslems listening with the closest attention, that we Genevan Protestants are, I think, particularly close to them, because Calvin bequeathed to us a keen sense of the immeasurable greatness of God.

Nevertheless, this consciousness of the distance between God and man leads Islam into fatalism, a passive form of acceptance. Our Christian piety, on the other hand, is nourished by our intimacy with Jesus. That is not to deny or forget the distance, since it was God, and not we, who crossed it in Jesus, and who thus knew the tensions of our human condition. Anyway, for me it is the intimacy with Jesus which commits me to active acceptance, because it is in suffering that I especially perceive his nearness, his presence, his participation in my life. I believe we can face everything when we believe we are loved.

The knowledge that we are loved is a potent factor too in coming to a calm and peaceful acceptance, rather than the tense acceptance of the stoics. The latter has its grandeur. Like ours, it is opposed to the passivity of resignation and fatalism. But it is a gritting of the teeth, and involves a certain hardening of attitudes – or, to put it in psychological terms, the repression of sentiment and tenderness, which are regarded as weakness.

The stoic aspires to emotional insensibility in order the better to stand firm in adversity. But the price to be paid is a stiffness which is quite different from the attitude of Jesus. We are told that he wept at the news of the death of his friend Lazarus (John 11.35). He is all tenderness towards those who are suffering adversity, and shares their emotion. I have often detected among my patients, especially among those who are Protestants, a whiff of stoicism in their attitude: men who will not allow themselves to weep, or women ashamed of their emotions. Dr Dubois of Berne used to praise what he called Christian stoicism. It has indeed forged strong personalities, as witness the rebellion of the Camisards. Nevertheless Calvin, in spite of his austerity, was very sensitive, capable of touching friendships and of great tenderness, as Jean-Daniel Benoît has shown in his book on Calvin as a pastor.

You can see how the problem of acceptance is a tangle of all kinds of factors, not only religious and philosophical, but also psychological, relating to childhood experiences, as well as constitutional, hereditary, and genetic factors. The whole of my career as a doctor has taught me that the question is too complicated to allow of any simplistic pronouncement. There are fervent believers who find it exceedingly difficult to accept the slightest disappointment or mishap, while there are un-believers to whom acceptance comes without great difficulty. The believers tend to blame themselves for lack of faith, and engage in an impotent struggle with themselves, the result of which is to aggravate their nervous state and their fear of having judgment passed upon them by others, despite their trust in God's love and forgiveness. It is a tragic vicious circle!

The same vicious circle frequently operates when parents blame themselves for their nervous irritation with a child who will not stop crying. The more irritated they become, the more the child cries; and the more the child cries, the more upset they are. Even trying to control themselves and quieten the child by means of kisses only makes matters worse, for the child is quite capable of reading the unconscious minds of his parents and seeing there the anger that is hidden behind their tactical tenderness. We must remember that acceptance is impossible for the very small child: he can only smile when his needs are satisfied, and weep at the slightest deprivation. He can also feel his parents' preference for a brother or sister, despite their denials – and it is natural: it is so easy to handle a child who smiles and redoubles his smiles at every embrace. Inevitably there are deprivations and vicious circles in the business of living together as a family. Freud, who had listened to so many accounts of them, made this comforting comment: 'In bringing up children, whatever you do is wrong.'

Nevertheless, however difficult the tangle of psychological reactions, it seems obvious to me that religious faith is the most powerful source of real acceptance. No doubt you have known or read of striking examples of this: disabled people, or the victims of cruel deprivations, who not only know peace, but radiate joy to all around them, because of their experience of faith. I am thinking now of a French friend of mine, Suzanne

Fouché – of her book *Souffrance, école de vie*, and also of the work she does.

An intelligent and active girl, she was intending to study medicine, but was struck down in adolescence by an insidious disease which soon revealed itself as tuberculosis of the bone. It was to confine her to bed in one sanatorium after another over a period of eighteen years. She hides neither her early despair nor her early rebellion, nor yet the painful problems and struggles that her disease has constantly imposed upon her. But the 'yes' that she was able to pronounce, and which was to sustain her and to grow in her life, was much more a 'yes' to God than to her disease, which she has never stopped fighting.

While she was still young, and still in the sanatorium, she saw how enforced idleness damaged the morale of the inmates and vitiated their treatment. One by one she drew them towards her with this simple admonition, which I myself now repeat to my old people: 'Do what you can!' In this way she organized from her sick-bed small groups engaged in every possible kind of activity. The movement spread, and became a league which transformed the lives of more and more sick people. The organization grew, and spreading beyond the world of the sick it became an enormous charity which gradually set up Homes for the rehabilitation of physically handicapped people. There are now more than thirty such Homes throughout France.

There is one near Geneva, at Evian. When I heard about it I wanted to see it. In the bank one day I took the opportunity of asking the cashier if he could tell me the right address. His face lit up at once: 'I should just think I do know it,' he exclaimed, 'I owe everything to it!' He was one of Suzanne Fouché's miraculous successes. Heart disease had put a stop to his career, but in the Fouché Home he had been able to take up the study of accountancy, and had been able to lead a normal life at the bank. Suzanne Fouché follows the principle of giving the handicapped person a course of retraining which means for him a step up the social ladder, and access to a better life. There are thousands and thousands of people like that all over France.

It is a grand illustration of the link between deprivation and creativity. Suzanne Fouché's life has been far more creative and fruitful than if she had been able to become a doctor. In international conferences on the medicine of the person all my colleagues come to her, full of veneration, seeking inspiration for their own work. She is able to help them to see more clearly into the problems that weigh upon their patients, problems of which doctors are often unaware – for she has been an invalid all her life. But she can also bear witness to her faith, and to the creative personal contact which it brings about between doctor and patient.

7

Courage

This story prompts me to reply to a question which has probably been in your mind for some time as you read this book: what can we do to help the victims of some misfortune or deprivation to discover within themselves, by means of the very deprivation itself, fresh creative energy? My reply is: by communicating that sort of courage to them. Suzanne Fouché offers the physically handicapped an opportunity. They must go through a period of retraining; they are taught a trade; there is a well-thought-out technical organization in an appropriate setting. But what is also required is the thing that takes place inside them – the reawakening of their courage, without which the great effort at readaptation will not succeed. To provide them with the tool is fundamental; but they must also be given the necessary courage. This brings us back to what I have called the two tasks of the doctor, one scientific, the other moral.

Life is beautiful, but it is hard for all human beings, very hard even for the majority. It is even harder in misfortune, in the face of deprivation. That requires a lot of courage. I stress the fact because I am well aware that it is something of which I have very little. My own courage revives when I come into contact with courageous people – often my patients, more handicapped than I am, and displaying courage which I admire. For courage is not taught, it is caught. Society is a vast laboratory of mutual encouragement. Each member can give the other only the courage he has himself – doctors as well as patients.

Last week a female relative of mine who devotes herself to sick-visiting suddenly asked me: 'Don't you ever fail? Reading your books, one gets the feeling that you always find the right thing to say to everyone!' I laughed, but rather uneasily. Do I really give such a false picture of myself? I remembered there and then one of my most painful failures, the suicide of one of my patients who had become a close friend to me. That is what a doctor's life is. I thought of several of my doctor friends who suddenly discovered that a wife or a son was suffering from a cancer that was too far advanced for there to be any hope of a cure. Of others who had lost a child in some stupid accident, or who had had to watch a member of their family die in prolonged agony. That needs courage!

Last year I was asked to give a paper in a seminar on geriatry, on the subject of 'morale in old age'. I was convalescing at the time, and had plenty of time to prepare my talk. For such a learned audience I should of course have liked to produce original and interesting ideas. But even after weeks of racking my brains all that came into my head was 'Morale means courage! Morale means courage!' Nevertheless I had to find the courage to take the plunge with that rather modest offering as a jumping-off point. In the event it turned out to have a lot more to it than I had imagined.

We have all, in fact, a natural tendency to confuse 'morale' with 'optimism', to think that in order to sustain morale we have most of all to keep up the patient's hope that he is going to get well, or at any rate to improve in the near future. That is all right in the case of a short illness, when the patient can be told definitely from what he is suffering, that his disease is a well-known one, as is the treatment also, and even how long it will be before he is cured. Morale is not a great problem in such cases, unless there are family or business worries. It is quite a different matter in the many cases of chronic illness – in which morale is an important factor in the progress of the disease – and especially in the case of old age, which is not a disease but a normal and inevitable process.

The situation is then a complex one; there are chances and risks, joyful signs and alarming signs, possible ameliorations and retrogressions, which have to be accepted. In our eagerness to sustain our patients' optimism we naturally tend to present the balance-sheet in the most favourable light, minimizing the bad things and emphasizing the more hopeful factors: 'Yes, this ankylosis makes walking difficult for you; but you see, with the help of your walking-stick you *have* managed to go the few steps down the street to get your newspaper, and that's good!' – 'Yes, your memory is not as good as it once was, but at your age memory isn't all that important any more.' – 'You are becoming hard of hearing, but your sight is still good, you can read, and that's a very precious thing!' It's really a dialogue between the deaf!

Of course it is not often that a doctor or an experienced sick visitor puts it in such simplistic terms, but there are a thousand ways, some subtler than others, in which basically the same tactic is employed, even without our realizing it. It is, however, a sterile proceeding. The more the patient complains, the more we do it, and the harder we try to cheer him up, the more he complains. The reason is that he feels we are not understanding his situation and how much he is suffering. Only by acknowledging his suffering can we arouse in him courage sufficient to cope with his suffering. Through recognizing how hard it is to accept, we help him to accept.

Is it not really we ourselves who lack the courage, when we are more afraid than our patient of facing the truth? Because the truth is that our impotence, humiliating as it is for us, prompts us to run away from the dialogue of truth even more readily than he does. Morale is above all things courage, and the patient's courage depends on ours. Consider, for instance, the courage the drug-addict needs in order to free himself from his addiction; but how much courage is needed too by those who want to give him the support he requires.

Our job as doctors is a continual challenge to us, as Balint has pointed out, and that too demands courage. Elisabeth Kubler-Ross tells of how the first time she made up her mind to talk to a dying man in order to find out from him what his feelings were, she very soon found an excuse for putting it off until the next day. By then, of course, the man had died, and she realized that she had first to overcome her own fear of the emotion involved in such a dialogue. She shows us that it is we, who are well, who lack the courage to enter into such conversations. Even when we do we avoid asking the patient the questions we intended, and instead talk to him about other things, on the grounds that we have to distract him in order to keep up his morale.

It is the times of greatest trial that arouse the greatest courage. Winston Churchill galvanized the whole of Britain into action in 1940 by offering only blood, toil, tears, and sweat. It was the exact opposite of forced optimism; but it was indeed his own courage which he was communicating to others. We can see it clearly in such heroic circumstances. But we too often forget it when a sick or aged person brings his daily complaints, possibly minor ones, to which we find it easy to reply comfortingly that it is nothing very serious, not realizing that this is his own way of putting into words a much deeper anguish, heroic in its way, about the acceptance of ill-health, of old age, and of the possibility of death, the threat of which is constantly there in the background, whether or not he is conscious of it.

The necessary courage comes only with the trial itself. There are people who constantly worry over whether they will have the courage to face this or that deprivation – old age, a painful illness, infirmity, or the death of husband or wife. I have always tried to reassure them, for as long as the trial they fear is not there, the courage cannot be there either. And they are probably the ones who will bear it most courageously if it does come. Over and over again I have marvelled at the resources of courage these worrying people reveal themselves to have when they have to face the real thing and not the fantom of their imagination!

There is more to be said. There is the joy of which I have already spoken, that extraordinary joy which radiates from many a sufferer from serious infirmity, and which contrasts astonishingly with the moroseness of so many of the healthy people one sees on the bus. What is the explanation? Well, I think that it is because their lives demand permanent courage, a constant expenditure of courage; and since courage belongs to the spiritual economy, the more one spends it, the more one has. It is like a current flowing through them and producing joy, the joy of victory over one's fate. This joy in victory is something we find in all those who accomplish a great exploit – in the climber who reaches the summit of the Eiger via the north face; and in every champion in sport, even if they do collapse in tears of exhaustion at the winning-post. Moreover, in a seriously disabled person it is not the victory of a single day, but of every day. Where does the pleasure in living come from? More from struggling than from possessing.

The first time I spoke on this theme of deprivation was at a meeting of the Association of Single Mothers. The audience consisted therefore entirely of women who were widows, divorced or abandoned wives, or unmarried mothers, in charge of fatherless children and responsible for their upbringing. What I had to say to them about orphans could be an encouragement for them. But they did not need encouragement: I was struck by the joy that reigned among them. I reflected that they too had to expend plenty of courage each day in lives as hard as theirs, and the secret of their impressive joy was in that current of spiritual energy running through them. But there was also the phenomenon of communication – courage passing from one to the other; each drawing courage from the realization of the courage of the others, and contributing her own courage to that of the rest. It was like the multiplication of reflections in a hall of mirrors.

The most encouraged of all was myself. I came away from that meeting full of joyfulness, and when the organizer brought me a rose bush for my garden I felt that she deserved it more than I. It is very clear that nothing arouses in us more courage than meeting a man, woman, or child who is showing exemplary courage in adversity. It is far more effective than exhortation. It seems to me most important to emphasize this contagious quality of courage. For I see so many good people who try genuinely to resist all kinds of temptations out of faithfulness to their ideals, but who feel quite powerless in face of the fearful contagion of evil, of violence, injustice, and lies which is attacking the world. What can they do about it? Their daily obedience, worthy though it be, seems no more than a tiny drop lost in a stormy ocean. The contagion of good is not so obvious. However, one thing that is unmistakeable is the contagious effect of an exceptionally courageous obedience.

I can witness to the truth of this because I have experienced it. I have mentioned the decisive influence that was exercised on my life by the Oxford Group Movement. That movement was born out of an example of courageous obedience. An American minister, Frank Buchman, who was the director of an institute, had had a serious disagreement with his committee of management, and had been dismissed. Feeling extremely bitter, he had gone into a little chapel, and there in the silence he felt he was being called not only to forgive the members of the committee, but also to acknowledge his own fault, and to ask forgiveness of each one of them in a personal letter.

That is a very rare thing indeed. People the world over are ready to denounce the faults of others. And the others – what do they do? They always reassure themselves by denouncing in their turn the faults of others. It is a universal and permanent chorus of outraged criticism, blame, and accusation, going from man to man, group to group, party to party, nation to nation, all around the globe. It takes courage to face the struggle of life, to hold one's own against one's adversaries, even to kill one's enemies in war – and there, from the acts of heroism that take place, one can see clearly the contagious power of courage – but it also takes courage to recognize ourselves for what we are, to acknowledge not just 'our sins' in a generalized way, as we do rather glibly in the liturgy, but our quite concrete and shameful acts of wrongdoing, and to ask to be forgiven by someone for an injury we have quite personally done him.

I want to stress this fundamental distinction which I am making between our daily obedience to our duty, and other specific acts of obedience which demand exceptional courage. I am not belittling the former which of course is indispensable, and without which social life is impossible; but that sort of obedience is as it were a routine virtue, the result of a good upbringing. Even confession can lose its liberating efficacy when it lapses into routine. It is the exceptional gesture which takes us by surprise. I think that is what Jesus meant in the Sermon on the Mount. Jaspers pointed out that if we try to treat it as a moral code, as many people think of it, it turns out to be impossible to apply. To go two miles, for example, with whoever asks us to go one, is not feasible. Jesus himself on occasions refused what was asked of him.

The isolated, quite unexpected gesture prompted by love or by a sense of justice, never fails to be profoundly moving. I have told of how my classics master, when I was sixteen, transformed my shy, withdrawn orphan's life by inviting me to his home. I did not realize it at the time, but everything was changed for me from that day, because he was no longer acting professionally as a teacher towards his pupil, but personally towards me as a person. Thus the medicine of the person does not call for change in the professional routine we have learnt at medical school, whereas just a glance, an unexpected remark, or an unusual course of action, changes our relationship with the patient because he feels that he is not being looked upon merely as a case, but as a person.

I am reminded of a woman whose parents had brought her into the world as a replacement for a beloved daughter whom they had lost. She felt that she was not herself, but a sort of stand-in. Her illnesses and her personality troubles seemed to be manifestations of an unconscious search for her identity as a person. The same applied to her whims: she had a passion for fur coats, which she kept piled up in a cupboard without ever wearing them. She went out less and less. And so, instead of interviewing her in her home, I took her out for rides in the car; we went out often. I remember another, whom I had told that I was very fond of her, and she replied in a flash, 'It's all one to me, because you love everybody, don't you?' She was wrong, of course. You can't love everybody – and if you did, you would not love anyone. The love that doctors have for their patients does not suffice. The patient needs something more personal. It is always the exceptional which gets through.

So I come back to the story of Frank Buchman. It spread like wildfire among the students of Oxford University. One after another found, as if by a miracle, the courage to put his own life in order, to admit his faults and put them right, to dedicate his life to Jesus Christ. And joy broke out. It was a true example of the creativity which can burst out of misfortune. It is also an illustration of what we have together established, that it was not the trouble that Frank Buchman had gone through, which itself opened the floodgates to this torrent of creativity, but his courageous response to it. And courage is catching; and it grows like an avalanche, which once started rapidly gathers momentum. From its beginnings in Oxford the Movement spread to every country, and caught me up in my turn, thanks to a patient of my friend Dr Mentha, whom I had also treated, and the mysterious change in whom aroused our curiosity.

I was soon making a series of approaches myself towards reconciliation, as a result of remembering past conflicts during my times of meditation. Most of these conflicts had taken place within the church, even with my own pastor when we were both members of the Consistory. Years have gone by, full of overwhelming experiences which transformed our home life as well as that of so many people around us. Husbands and wives in conflict rediscovered harmony and mutual confidence; unbelievers found faith; unworthy actions were confessed and reparation made: a veritable epidemic of courage.

When it came to my patients, I realized that there was a dimension in medicine which I had not recognized. Insomniacs recovered the ability to sleep without medication, bulimics found they could control their appetite, hypertension and rheumatism sufferers found relief, dysmenorrhea disappeared. So many people go from one treatment to another – with some improvement, it is true, but such success as they have is precarious, for when one thing improves, other troubles appear. The fact is that the causes lie deeper; sometimes they are psychological, but also sometimes spiritual, arising out of their over-all attitude to life and to everything that has soured it for them. Illich has shown how medication and technical medicine generally may provide an easy means of avoiding more difficult decisions. As Sarano remarks, he makes a distinction, as it were, between 'courage-health' and 'comfort-health'.

A radical change can bring with it personal authenticity and a quite new health. This is why in his clinic in Germany my friend Dr Walther Lechler has actually given up all symptomatic medication, so that the patient when he enters may begin a new life free of artifice, become himself, express his feelings without constraint, find a meaning in his life and a true personal fellowship with other people. It demands a lot of courage, from patients as well as doctors.

I had a like experience myself nearly half a century ago. For my part, I did not renounce classical medicine. I sought to initiate myself into the techniques of psychology in order to embody them into my practice. One must not forget, however, that the scientific attitude is always objective and analytical. It recognizes only parts, organs, functions, psychological mechanisms; never the whole, the complete person, approachable only by committing oneself subjectively in relationship. It is precisely to this that spiritual communion leads the way; and that is the way I took, as did many others of my colleagues. Dr Theodore von Leiber had for a number of years been treating a woman for anaemia without ever achieving a haemoglobin count of more than 65%. Suddenly he found that it was over 80%! He asked her what had happened since her last visit, and was told that she too had found faith.

The movement was spreading, winning over doctors, theologians, politicians, people not much given to sentimental enthusiasms, on account of their education, their critical sense, and their position in society. But it was not confined to people in these privileged walks of life. Frida Nef, for instance, arrived in Lausanne from her home in the mountains like a waif, after a terrible childhood spent amidst poverty, shame, and over-work, because her father was an alcoholic. Finding faith she also found the courage to forgive him, and then, liberated from her bitterness, the courage to open – without money – a hostel for young women whom she drew into her astounding adventure. Almost half a century later she wrote the story of her life, but was hesitant about seeking publication. I urged her to do so, for such a simple account seemed to me to be so convincing. And now she is astonished to be in such demand as a speaker, to have so many readers of her book writing to thank her for the new courage it has given them. Martyrs throughout the ages have borne clear witness to the courage faith can inspire, and to how their courage can inspire our faith.

I tell you all this because I have lived through it myself. But the same phenomenon has occurred throughout history. It has always been the courageous obedience of one single person to God's call that has set in motion a powerful spiritual movement, whether it has been St Francis of Assisi, St Teresa of Avila, Martin Luther, John Wesley, William Penn, to name but a few. Obviously this is not the exclusive privilege of Christianity. Think of the far-reaching effects of the courage of the Buddha, of Socrates or of Demosthenes, of Mahomet or of Gandhi. If there is one single virtue that we all admire, it is courage.

Therein lies also the danger; for the contagious power of courage is the same when it is inspired not by God, but by hate or pride. Think of the courage of Hitler, which captivated so many naïve Germans when he defied the nations which had humiliated their country between the two world wars. That is why he was just as naïve himself in exhorting people to be courageous, without at the same time teaching them to listen to God.

Actually, I do not think we should ever be exhorting people to be courageous. To be really fruitful, courage must come spontaneously, in answer to an inner call. I can think of several women who have had the courage to give up the idea of divorce in circumstances in which it would have been justifiable. I would not have taken it upon myself to encourage them because it was they, and not I, who had to face the sufferings that their decision imposed upon them. Jesus puts us on our guard against placing upon others burdens which we do not bear ourselves (Luke 11.46).

I have always observed that when it is God who calls us to make that sort of decision he also gives us the strength to bear the consequences. And though it cannot be denied that divorce is contagious, marital fidelity is equally infectious.

In the perspective of this book, I must now return to my own situation as an orphan. I have just referred to the part played by my classics master. I was, however, still incapable of expressing my repressed emotions. So what was it that suddenly gave me the courage to do so? Well, it was the courage of a Dutch civil servant, a senior official in the League of Nations, who also invited me to his house, and who dared to talk quite concretely about his faults. What took place was the communication of courage.

For while there is a universal network for the communication of courage, rather similar to the circulation of the blood in the organism, carrying oxygen to the tiniest cell, there is, closely related to it, also a communications network for the emotions. We men are even more afraid of our emotions than women; and not only of our own emotions and of the added emotion aroused in ourselves by our expressing them, but also of the emotions of others, which in turn arouse added emotion in us when they express them! It takes courage therefore to show our emotions – with the possible exception of anger – and it takes courage likewise to accept the emotions of others. That is why, in our Western world, most people stick carefully to intellectual discussion and objective theorizing, which do not require us to involve anything of ourselves or of our personal emotions. And it is also the reason why we are so lonely with our unexpressed emotions. The communication of courage and that of the emotions go hand in hand, and are the necessary condition of personal contact.

A Basle publisher named Reinhardt had the idea of producing a book composed of a chapter from each of my books, carefully chosen by Dr Charles de Roche. He needed a title and he chose *Mutig leben* (Living Courageously). And when a theologian, Monroe Peaston, wrote a book as an introduction to my work, he gave it the title *Personal Living*. The putting together of these two titles is a good illustration of the fact that in my eyes courage in face of the difficulties of life and personal contact are clearly connected. I think this is true of all psychotherapists, for there is no effective cure without moments of intense emotion – emotional discharge for the patient and emotional charge for the doctor, who in order to help his patient courageously accepts, and thus communicates courage to the patient.

This is also the case with the telephone 'helpline' services, which in Switzerland are given the name 'Helping Hand', and which respond to the terrible loneliness of our time that I have just referred to. To my mind that must be even more difficult than psychotherapy, because the respondent has to confine himself to listening – a role which is even more passive and less technical than that of the doctor. And then the telephone Samaritan is not able to plead the tyranny of the clock, as we can in our surgeries, much to our patients' chagrin. What courage it must take never to put the 'phone down before the caller himself terminates the communication! I admire those who devote themselves to this work, especially since I do not like the telephone – it lacks eye-contact, and telephone silences, silences which in a *tête-à-tête* are invaluable, are soon turned to anguish. That is why I am dedicating this book to Dr Klaus Thomas who introduced the service to Europe, and to Pastor Raynald Martin, who started it in Switzerland.

Whoever wishes to help others courageously to bear their misfortunes must accept the emotional charge which is involved in listening attentively, *empathetically*, as Carl Rogers says. There exists a continual traffic from person to person, as each discharges his own emotional burden on to the other as he expresses to him his anger, his misfortunes, and his despair. Our privilege as Christians is our ability in our turn to interrupt this chain-reaction by laying our burden on Jesus in the intimacy of our daily communication with him. He himself invited us to do so, and I am always experiencing the reality of it. In his company I can lay down the burden of the emotions which others have brought to me. Not enough, I know! My wife and I came to realize one day that we had a tendency to have an argument in the evening when during the day I had been helping to reconcile other couples. It was as if the demon that had come out of them had entered into me. Happily we were able to pray about it together.

It is also in Jesus that I can find courage, for he is the pattern of all courage, as everybody accepts. He was most courageous in his obedience to the Father. Even unbelievers, without knowing it, lay their burdens on him through our intermediary. The professors at the Islamic Faculty of Theology in Teheran questioned me about the Christian cure of souls. I answered that in my view it was essentially a ministry of reconciliation of man with himself and with God, of confession and absolution. For it is on coming to Jesus that each of us finds the courage to recognize ourselves for what we are, and then to accept ourselves because we are accepted, pardoned, and loved by Jesus just as we are. We talked about this at great length, because it implied an individual self-awareness which, they said, was rare in Islam. John the Baptist preceded Jesus to prepare the way for him (Matt. 3.3). Thus it is confession which opens the way to adhesion – the word used by André Chouraqui, a Jew, to express faith in Jesus Christ, in his fine translation of the New Testament.

The courage to be true to oneself, instead of allowing oneself to be contaminated by all the compromises of society. Alexander Solzhenitsyn denounces the decline in courage in our modern world. That was one of the main themes of his speech to the students at Harvard in 1978. He told those young Americans what they already knew – that he fought against the system in power in his own country; but he went on: 'I could not recommend your society as an ideal for the transformation of ours.' He added: 'A decline in courage may be the most striking feature that an outside observer notices in the West today.' Liberty in the West has become no more than 'almost unlimited freedom in the choice of pleasures'. The only concern is the preservation of unjust privileges: 'there must be no changes'.

He proposes to seek the mistake 'at the root, at the very foundation of thought in modern times . . . born in the Renaissance . . . it could be called rationalistic humanism'. 'Subsequently . . . a total emancipation occurred from the moral heritage of Christian centuries with their great reserves of mercy and sacrifice.' He asserts that we have been 'deprived of our most precious possession: our spiritual life. It is trampled by the party mob in the East, by the commercial one in the West.' I do not recall who it was who compared Solzhenitsyn with Galileo: Galileo had the courage to uphold reason in a world dominated by unreason, and Solzhenitsyn has the courage to uphold the irrational in a world that is exclusively rational.

Is not this decline in courage the price paid for prosperity in our privileged Western countries, for the 'deprivation of deprivation' of which I wrote at the beginning of this book? I am reminded of a conversation with Paul Ricoeur. He was asking me what I thought was the root cause of all the problems of life brought to me in my consulting-room. I answered, 'lack of courage'. He seemed surprised, and said rather sharply, 'Give me an example!' I quoted the first example that came into my mind – the marital conflicts which take up so much of my own and my colleagues' time. When one looks more closely into them, one sees that they have been latent for years, but that the couple did not have the courage to enter into a truthful dialogue together at the time when they were happy and in love. Now they are both horrified at the torrent of mutual complaints that pours out when the dam behind which they have been shut away suddenly bursts. They had thought that they were doing the right thing in keeping them back and so safeguarding their happiness and their love, when it was really lack of courage.

Why is courage necessary in misfortune? First, because in facing it courageously we suffer far less than if we lapsed into despair. Everybody knows that, including those who lack courage, and who would dearly like to be more courageous in order to suffer less. Unfortunately, the will is not enough. When we try to encourage a person suffering from depression, he always thinks that we are appealing to his will, which he feels to be too weak, and this further discourages him. His reaction, too, in the face of a courageous example is the opposite of ours. He is simply persuaded that what is possible for others is not possible for him, and he loses courage instead of finding it. We must understand him so that he will feel himself to be understood; we must understand that it is actually his sickness, and not lack of will-power, which is depriving him of courage.

For a healthy person, every trial is easier to bear if he can shoulder it courageously. But more important still is the result of this attitude, namely creativity. I must return to the point now, since it was this mysterious connection between deprivation and creativity which moved me to write this book. Remember that the work of Dr Rentchnick and of Dr Haynal has shown us that the majority of creative minds – politicians, religious leaders, philosophers, scientists, writers, and artists – have suffered much more than others from frustration and deprivation; and that this phenomenon may be observed not only in the life of individuals, but also in that of nations.

We have got to the point of wondering if suffering is really fruitful, as is sometimes affirmed; wondering even if it is sent by God among men for their own good, as some have thought. We have rejected this sophism, but we have concluded that while suffering may not be creative in itself, we are scarcely ever creative without suffering. As the idea of creativity involves to a greater or less degree those of growth and development, one could also say that it is not suffering which makes a person grow, but that one does not grow without suffering; again, that all deprivation and all suffering are opportunities for creativity. It remains for us to try to understand better why this is so.

8

Noise, *in the* Theory *of* Information

It was the reading of a book which for me threw an exciting
new light on the problem. I should like to share my excitement
with you. It was a book by a doctor, Henri Atlan, a professor
of biophysics, entitled *Entre le cristal et la fumée; essai sur
l'organisation du vivant.* You know what a large number of inventions and technical developments have resulted over the last
three decades from new disciplines: data processing, the theory
of information formulated by C. E. Shannon in 1948 to meet
the requirements of telecommunications, and cybernetics or
the possibility of governing, that is of making decisions, in
accordance with information received. Combined with electronics, they have made possible the pocket calculator and the
computer, inventions which are changing our life-style.

I wonder if the amazing development of the computer is
related solely to its usefulness. Perhaps it is due in part to the
fascination that mechanical toys have for children of all ages –
including grown men! It has become an indispensable tool of
scientific research; even more, these new disciplines have transformed scientific thought itself. And not only in the natural
sciences and in their teaching in universities, but also in philosophy and even theology – a point which Bernard Morel was
quick to grasp. As long ago as 1964 his remarkable book

entitled *Cybernétique et transcendance* was published.

It is, however, especially biology which has been directed into new avenues and new methods. The smallest reflex corresponds exactly to the model of the theory of information, with its two messages, the one sensory and the other motor, each consisting of the same succession: entry-coding-decoding-exit. The whole of the nervous system functions in accordance with this model. The analogy with the computer is striking, despite the enormous difference in the number of connections, since the human brain contains ten billion neurons – a figure beyond the dreams of the manufacturers of computers. There are other differences, of course, but they are not at all of the same order. I heard Dr Jean de Rougemont say once, 'Yes, the brain is a sort of computer, but it asks itself a question which no computer will ever ask: "What on earth am I doing here?" '

The main difference between the computer and the automatic machine of the living being is, as Henri Atlan has pointed out, a fundamental one. It is that the living machine manufactures itself and gives itself its programme, whereas a computer can never be anything more than its constructor has made it, and can follow only the programme of its operator. Atlan asks whether biology may not make a contribution to the perfecting of the computer, in exchange for the progress that cybernetics has brought to biological science, especially in the field of organization.

It is not only a matter of the nervous system. Each of the estimated thirty billion cells in our body receives and transmits information, encoding what it sends out and decoding what comes in. The discovery of the genetic code has brought striking proof that nature functions in accordance with the theory of information, as Madame Andrée Goudot-Perret has shown. Indeed, the genes, which occur in the chemical form of large DNA molecules, control the synthesis of the proteins, which in turn determine all the characteristics and the morphological, physico-chemical, and functional structures of the organism. The whole system corresponds to the classic model of the theory of information. There are four kinds of DNA, according to their respective bases: A (Adenine), T (Thymine), G (Guanine), and C (Cytosine), which through their grouping in successive sequences (triplets or codons) constitute a coded message 'written in an alphabet of four symbols', the whole being conveyed in the binary language of the computer.

Furthermore, it is a universal system of information, 'since it consists of a method of coding which is common to all the living organisms so far studied'. It thus ensures the stability of species through the faithful communication of the message from generation to generation, and, in the interior of each organism, from cell to cell. To crown all, it has been possible to decipher the code, just as Champollion deciphered that of Egyptian hieroglyphics, and to draw up a table of the triplets corresponding to each one of the twenty nucleic acids.

Henri Atlan's chief preoccupation, as I have said, is one day perhaps to discover the key to biological organization – in other words, the secret of life. Because living things are composed of the same atoms as the inorganic world. There are said to be 7×10^{27} (that is 7 followed by 27 noughts!) atoms in the adult human body. Consequently we must be made up of the same kind of atomic particles as those which the nuclear physicists at the European Research Centre in Geneva, or in the United States, or in Russia, produce by accelerating atoms to fantastic speeds in their circular tunnels, and then smashing them to pieces against their screens. So the living thing is not distinguishable from the inorganic world in respect of its composition, but only in its organization, and it is the secret of this that is sought by biophysicists such as Henri Atlan.

What an exciting adventure that is! I wasted no time before

reading a more comprehensive book by this same research scientist: *L'organisation biologique et la théorie de l'information.* Of course I did not understand all about the algorithms of equations – I have done no maths for more than sixty years, apart from the odd mathematical teaser in the puzzle corner of the newspaper, which I always enjoy doing. But I was keen enough on mathematics still to find considerable pleasure in trying to understand such sciences as data processing, cybernetics, and electronics, all of them unknown when I was a student. In any case, I find it very enjoyable, whereas there are lots of old people of my age who are bored, and never think of filling in the gaps in their knowledge. You see how my creativity is stimulated by the things I have missed! As William the Silent said, 'It is not necessary to hope in order to undertake, nor is success necessary to perseverance'.

I did not need to understand all of Atlan's equations, because my preoccupation was different from his – not the elucidation of the mystery of biological organization, but the problem of creativity resulting from deprivation. I at once saw what it was that the theory of information could contribute, through the new notion of 'noise'.

What is it that Shannon's theory calls noise? There are two ways in which it may be illustrated. When I am telephoning, and the line is good, communication is excellent, and I understand my caller perfectly. But if the line is defective there are extraneous noises which interfere with communication, and I have difficulty in understanding what is being said. The second illustration is the minute attention with which a mechanic listens to a machine running, ready to detect the slightest unusual sound which will betray some fault, and allow him to diagnose it, rather like the doctor listening to his patient's heart and lungs. Here then is what Atlan writes: 'Errors in transmission are produced by various factors which intervene in a random manner, and which are therefore called noise factors.'

Shannon developed his theory with a view to getting maximum efficiency in telecommunications. As Atlan says, his theory is concerned only with the efficient transmission of the message, like a postal service, paying no regard to its content. From this standpoint, of course, noise factors were looked upon as enemies which must be fought with all possible means, by repetition of the text, by ingenious forms of coding, and by other techniques. But with the application of the theory of information to biology we witness an astonishing turn-around: all at once the enemy may be seen as an ally and friend! Noise, otherwise so damaging, can have a 'beneficial effect', Atlan writes, picking up Weaver's expression. We must now examine this paradox.

There is in the first place the evolution of the species. You know that Darwin's theory has been challenged, despite its plausibility, because it involved the hereditary transmission of acquired characteristics. In fact this transmission has never been observed, a point that is better understood now, since the discovery of the genetic code, which obviously remains unaffected by all the vicissitudes which the subject may encounter during the course of its life. De Vries rehabilitated transformism by his idea of sudden, spontaneous mutations, infrequent enough to elude any forecast. All biologists now accept this so-called neo-transformist theory.

But of course De Vries' mutations correspond precisely to Atlan's definition of noise: random errors in the transmission of the code. And while one may find it impossible to conceive of the hereditary transmission of acquired characteristics, there is no difficulty in accepting the possibility of the transmission of a deformed code. So, then, it is noise – that is to say, a succession of random errors in the duplication of the code – which is the necessary and sufficient key to the whole evolution of species, from unicellular organisms right up to man, demonstrating fantastic progression in complexity. We may well speak, therefore, of the 'beneficial effect' of noise!

There is, however, more to it still. The fact is that this progression in complexity, in the anatomical, physiological, and psychological differentiation which is characteristic of the living world, its organization – in short, its order – would appear to proceed from noise. That is Henri Atlan's thesis, the fruit of his own work, following upon that of Von Foerster, who was the first to formulate the 'principle of order arising out of noise'.

Clearly we are here in the realm of hypothesis, and even though these are plausible ones, full of promise, they still require plenty of work to be done on them before they can be verified, and I am not competent to discuss them seriously. It is, however, fascinating to follow these biologists in their researches. What I derive from them is the new perspectives they open out for our own thought about good and evil, about misdeeds and benefits, about misfortunes and creativity. Noise is a fault, an evil. As we have seen, it compromises information. It must be combated. But it introduces a new element to be transmitted, and so may enrich the information. So that Atlan writes: 'It is possible and not contradictory that what appears as destruction of information when viewed in isolation, may be seen as the creation of information when viewed in the context of the whole.'

Does not that remind us of something? You remember Madame Monique Kressmann, who told us how destructive a slight disagreement with her husband had seemed at the time, but afterwards, when viewed in a wider perspective – that of the whole of life – it had seemed to her to be constructive. You must surely have already felt, as I did, that there is a striking analogy between the notion of noise in data-processing and that of deprivation which I have borrowed from Dr Haynal. Noise is a form of deprivation! The words themselves suggest the analogy: noise is an error in transmission, a deprivation of exactitude in the information, which makes it faulty. Faulty – there is a word which involves two kinds of meaning: deprivation as well as error.

But the analogy goes further. Noise is that which disturbs the transmission of information, upsetting the proper ordering of things, their normal course. And that is precisely the effect of all the kinds of deprivation of which I have spoken. A death – that of their parents in the case of Dr Rentchnick's orphans – an accident, a sickness, a failure, a disappointment in love, an infirmity, old age: and all at once the normal course of life is no longer possible. This it is that seriously affects us, like the noise which destroys information.

But listen to Atlan once again: 'If, under the action of these random disturbances the (organic) system, instead of being destroyed or disorganized, reacts in an increase of complexity and continues to function, we then say that the system is self-organizing ... In other words, the property of self-organization seems to be connected with the ability to use random disturbances – "noise" – in order to produce organization.' So you see, we are back once more to the dilemma of deprivation as I have described it, with its two possible reactions: destruction or creativity. And we are also back to the distinction on which I have insisted: it is not the noise itself which produces the creativity, but the reaction of the subject to the noise. Clearly, if the work of the biologists can explain for us what it is that tips the balance to the right side or to the wrong side, it would be an enormous help to us.

Marital conflicts, for example, which I have mentioned, and which Paul Plattner has so well described, are a good illustration of this process. Through a long series of tiny conflicts as the spouses adapt to each other, provided they face up to them courageously, there slowly develops a psychological organization of their life together which is at once more complex and more productive and solid than the simplistic relationship of the honeymoon. Whereas other couples, who do not have that courage, avoid the conflicts for the sake of peace, and as a result they become strangers to each other, and all kinds of repressed grudges can suddenly come to the surface, with catastrophic consequences.

When I read about the theory of information and the notion of noise, I could not but be reminded of those pedagogues whose only aim in life is to get a faultless exercise from a pupil, and who know no other means of assessing marks than counting up the mistakes he has made. Oh! It is not my purpose to attack professional teachers, for we are all the same. Which parents do not expect perfection from their children? One could paraphrase Beaumarchais' famous remark in *Le Barbier de Séville*: 'Judging from the virtues that are required of a child, does your Excellency know many parents who would be worthy of being children?'

I am reminded of a thought that came to me once, and which I have never dared to put into print. Listening to a neurotic telling me about his childhood, which had been as repressed as that of Fritz Zorn, to which I have already referred, I murmured: 'Woe betide the child who has never cheated.' I feared that I should be accused of preaching against the most basic morality, that of truthfulness. But what other means has the feeble child to defend himself against his almighty parents? Are not even the habits of animals full of ruses that are indispensable to their survival, as Dröscher has so clearly demonstrated? Happily, I cheated, just as all healthy children do. I slipped my Latin grammar under Fabre's *Souvenirs of a Naturalist* so as to be able quickly to replace it on top should I hear footsteps coming towards my room. That gave me some bad marks in Latin, but also a passionate interest in biology.

It is, however, possible to be over-exacting with oneself. I have treated numbers of so-called perfectionists whose lives have been paralysed by an obsessive fear of making the slightest mistake. Their fear had smothered every spark of creativity in them, because it can flourish only in the free air of spontaneity.

How consoling, therefore, it is to discover that it is through our mistakes that we grow! It is like a profane translation of the old religious adage, *Felix culpa*, the happy fault! How comforting it is to learn that it is probably through mistakes in copying the genetic code that there has developed the whole living world, including this prodigious being we call man, at which the psalmist invites us to marvel (Ps. 19). This then is God's method, God's pedagogy, the art of 'using random disturbances – noise – in order to produce organization': the words of Atlan which I quoted just now. The production of organization, is that not the very work of the Creator, in the eyes of the scientist as well as in those of the believer?

I incline to the belief that it is in fact God's method to use noise, to salvage noise, one might say, as Atlan shows, in order to realize his plan, just as he uses evil for our salvation. This is the refutation of the Manicheism which would oppose good (information free from noise) and evil (the noise which disturbs it). That is what happened on the cross, where the most unjust evil turns out to be the greatest blessing.

We psychotherapists have a name for noise, the spoiler, the random factor which disturbs information, we call it a lapse. Yes, of course – noise is a lapse of information! De Vries' unexpected mutation is also a lapse in the communication of the genetic code. Thus it is to lapses in DNA that we owe the wonderful diversity of living species. That is less surprising than it seems if we think of the role of lapses in the evolution of languages: how has one and the same word in Latin been transformed into three different words in Italian, French, and Spanish, except by a series of lapses?

A lapse in my speech betrays me; it hinders the communication of my thought. If I notice it, I hasten to excuse myself: 'Sorry! I am wrong!' So it is a fault, a deprivation. Proof of this is that Freud classified it as what he called a 'bungled action', along with lapses of memory, and all the disturbances in non-verbal language – gestures, conduct and manners that are unbefitting to the conscious intention.

Before Freud, lapses and all kinds of bungled actions were looked upon as no more than annoying accidents. The genius of Freud lay in the fact that he demonstrated that they were by no means accidental, but that they had a meaning, that they too were a language, a form of information, and of great importance. So that in speech there are two layers of information: one manifest, which the speaker wishes to communicate, and the other unconscious, expressing something quite different. The first is disturbed and diminished, but what the lapse reveals is added to it, so that the total of information conveyed is greater. This is precisely what Atlan says in the passage quoted on the subject of noise.

To whichever school they claim to belong, all psychologists are agreed on Freud's theory of 'bungled actions'. We too can constantly verify it in our daily practice. Thanks to Freud we can, generally speaking, easily decipher the meaning of a lapse; at least we can suspect it, both in our own lapses and in those of our patients (who, moreover, have a good idea of it themselves). An accident that has a meaning is no longer an accident. You will notice that Henri Atlan, unlike Jacques Monod, avoids the use of the word accident, preferring to speak of aleatory (i.e. unforeseeable) factors (*alea*, in Latin, means the throw of a dice). One can foresee a physical phenomenon because one knows its cause. A psychological phenomenon remains aleatory; but it can be understood afterwards, through its meaning, its purpose.

One thinks too of the errors made by the copyists in the transmission of ancient manuscripts through the centuries. They give trouble enough to students and men of letters. Of course they must first detect them in order to establish the authentic text. But they may also ask themselves why the copyist made the error, and the answer to that question is itself not without interest for literary history.

Although he denied it, notably in his controversy with Jung, Freud reintroduced the notion of purpose into science. But the geneticists have done the same, and so too has this theory of noise, for if noise is a lapse it has a meaning, a purpose! This too Atlan expressly says: 'A singular event arises to disturb communication in one of the channels of the system, and a meaning is born.'

Let us see, then, what can happen when a lapse takes place. It is fortunate that they do take place, since they reveal to us problems that we should otherwise not be able to detect. A man with the air of an overgrown schoolboy, who allows himself to be mothered by his wife, who leaves every responsibility to her, who blames her for all his present difficulties as if she should have protected him from them, makes a slip in talking about her, calling her 'Mummy' instead of 'My wife'. He can understand the truth expressed by this lapse much more readily than if the doctor had told him; for it is not a matter of the intellectual understanding of a theory, but of his feeling that this is the trouble he is suffering from – that he behaves like a baby, tyrannizing over his wife as an infant does over his mother, that he is anxious and jealous if she leaves him in order to live her own life. And it is not even this discovery which is the essential thing, but rather the road he must take that will make him able and keen to shoulder his adult responsibilities.

Of course I have over-simplified in this scenario a process that is nothing like so straightforward, nor is it without its dramatic moments. It could also arise from the analysis of a dream. But in this case it was in fact a lapse which triggered it off. He was quick to excuse his mistake as an accidental slip of the tongue, as if he were trying to avoid a deeper investigation. Among the believers I have treated, people quite convinced that God had a purpose for them, I have seen many who imagined they could fulfil it only through impeccable obedience, without committing the least error, so that it was almost a moral obsession with them. How comforting, then, to know that God also uses our faults to guide us.

Henri Atlan quotes my fellow-citizen Jean Piaget, whom I used to love to meet, and what Piaget calls learning without a teacher. There are two ways of learning: with or without a teacher. Of course a book is also a teacher. The teacher tells us what we must know and do in order to act properly, to count correctly, to speak or write effectively, to draw well, to sew neatly, to plane smoothly, to ski, and so on. We have to memorize it all in order to be able to do the thing correctly first time; and every mistake is penalized with a bad mark in order to re-awaken our memory. The other method is that of trial and error, which means feeling our way, on our own, for our own amusement, making countless trials and lots of errors, until we discover for ourselves how best to achieve: a ton of errors for an ounce of success!

It is this method which particularly pleases and suits children, whom Piaget studied so perceptively, children bursting with curiosity and creativity, who touch everything, handle everything, who love to try everything just to see what happens, not concerned to do it correctly, with none of the fear of making a mistake which is so paralysing to adults. This is how they discover the world and gradually adapt themselves to it; it is how they discover themselves, their possibilities and their limitations. When a child has succeeded in co-ordinating his movements sufficiently, which no teacher could have taught him, he moves forward, and we all exclaim, 'He's walking!' But he does not know that – he will need a teacher to tell him that what he has just done is called walking.

Of course his education must be completed by the other method, by a rigorously planned scholastic routine; but it will not have the same savour of personal creativity – it will give him more learning than knowledge. The teacher can teach me that Paris is on the Seine, Rome on the Tiber, and New York on the banks of the Hudson. But having actually been there I am reminded of walks along the embankments of the Seine, discussing the meaning of our vocation with an old friend, and turning over the pages of the old books in the picturesque bookstalls there; or the silhouette of the Castle of Sant'Angelo on the banks of the Tiber, or the great bridge over the Hudson. There! I have forgotten what it is called. I should have to look it up on the map! But as Foucault has pointed out, it is more important to know things than names. The map is indeed a thing, but an artificial one, which teaches all the names, but is not living. Nevertheless, in order to learn geography I had to submit myself to the routine of school.

So there are two complementary means of discovering the world. The quite spontaneous method of trial and error of the small child remains defective, discontinuous, hitty-missy like life itself. It proceeds bit by bit, making dots that are not connected by any line. It is attracted by the unique, the unusual, the interesting detail, and it marvels. The systematic method prefers the repetitive, it looks for laws, sets out parameters, constructs theories, and leads to erudition. It all depends on one's state of mind more than on what one does. There are people who travel in an entirely routine fashion, and poets who, like Klopfenstein, feel that 'the sun is new every day'.

9

Routine and Creativity

So there is a dialectic of the unique and the repetitive. The trial and error method exploits and stimulates creativity and the search for something new and unforeseeable; the other method institutes routine. Creativity is the truly new, unique, unforeseen fact. Routine repeats it immediately, and then it is no longer creativity for that very reason. Life is inconceivable without the new and unforeseen departure. The problem of the origin of life, Atlan says, has only been pushed back to that of the appearance of the first programme, since from that moment it will be reproduced unless there is a 'noise', marking a new departure. Thus routine is the fruit of life; but it is at the same time what deprives it of its peculiar character and petrifies it. Albert Delaunay in a published interview tells of a creative-minded student who wanted to do research in physics, and told his teacher of his desire. The latter replied that if he wanted to do research he ought to look elsewhere, because, he said, physics was complete, totally explored, so that there was no more research to be done. That student was Max Planck, who fortunately did stick to physics despite the disillusioned advice he had received; and he shook its foundations, roused it out of its lethargy, and brought it back to life with his quantum theory. It is a marvellous story. Physics, the most scientific of disciplines, was thus the one to rediscover the discontinuous, the random, the unforeseeable, of which all that we can measure is its probability.

Since Planck it is no longer possible to picture the electron always moving soberly on its elliptical orbit without cheating; instead it jumps from one orbit to another, and not in accordance with any set pattern, but skipping over in a way that I find utterly charming; especially since one cannot forecast the jump, but only the probability that it will happen. I too skip about, from science to religion, from genetics to psychoanalysis; and I tend to put out those systematic thinkers who keep reminding me that one ought not to mix the genres, as they say. I too have my little quantum of energy. It is minuscule, like all quanta, but it is my own, and it drives me where it wills, despite the dogmatisms of science, of religion, or of psychoanalysis. I do not mix them, I skip from one to the other, and that is what keeps me young. Curiosity always looks over the wall. I have made up a slogan on the subject for use in my talks on preparing for retirement: As long as you are curious you won't grow old!

The shaking of the foundations of physics and the quantum theory come to my assistance, as you see. These electrons skipping about instead of going round and round have an air of youth about them – even the so-called lone electrons, which jump about in search of the positive charge that will satisfy them. Gone now are the triumphant tones in which we used to be told in my student days about the absolute and universal determinism definitively demonstrated by science, which left no room for the notion that the world was created by God, and that man had been divinely endowed as a person with freedom and responsibility. I had already had the good fortune to be taught by Charles E. Guye, who was the first to give an experimental demonstration of Einstein's theory, and who insisted always on the statistical character of the laws of nature, so that their apparent rigour resulted from the fine individual fantasy of the dancing electrons and other such elementary particles.

At first sight our Western technological civilization would appear to favour creativity, since it has been the scene of so many marvellous discoveries and inventions. But that is an illusion. In reality it has reserved the adventure of creativity to a handful of privileged people – the scientists in their research laboratories and the powerful barons of industry. Outside them, it has transformed the vast mass of our contemporaries into robots or sheep whose life is nothing but an incredibly monotonous and tiring routine. The worker is lost in a gigantic organization performing a job that is a mere mechanical routine completely without interest, unless he is one of the few that are lucky enough to be very high up in the professional hierarchy.

When society relied on the craftsman, his personal creativity was constantly called upon. He had to improvise all sorts of things, often making his own tools, seeking ingenious and effective ways of solving the problems his craft presented. The craftsman created something out of nothing; he could see the result of his work, and sold it direct to the consumer, with the chance of a bit of conversation, even a bargaining session the conclusion of which each knew in advance, but it gave them the opportunity for a subtle little game and real personal contact. The craftsman could be encouraged by hearing at first hand the quality of his merchandise and his craftsmanship being praised; and he could hear the criticisms as well, and set about working out how to overcome in some original way the problems they raised. There were long fitting sessions at the dressmaker's, and cookery recipes to pass on. Now we get our ready-to-wear clothes from the hypermarket, along with the ready-made dish that goes straight from the freezer into the oven. The hum of the washing-machine has taken over from the chatter of the washerwomen. One used to meet one's friends in the street, where now all they get is a brief wave from a car.

That is still the way of life in what we call the developing countries, where they still make their own bread, thresh their own wheat, pluck their own chickens, and gossip endlessly in the square. What we have developed is only society, the collectivity, the organization, regimentation, planning, bureaucracy, economy, mechanics, and anonymous impersonal technology. As for man's need to be treated not as a machine for production but as a person, to assert his personal identity, and to have genuine relationships with other people, in short to live in conviviality (to use Illich's excellent term), we are incontestably under-developed – not even developing, but regressing.

Everything is sacrificed to profit and to material prosperity. If only it could ensure a living wage for the whole of humanity! But the West with all its scientists and all its machines has not achieved that. It would have the whole of the Third World on its side if it could do so. On the contrary, it turns out that our wealth depends on low-priced raw materials, on the poverty of others. If at the very least our material prosperity fostered culture! But culture has slipped away from the silence of the library, where there was a chance to sit down and think, into the racket of the media. Even our pleasures have become mass movements, radio-controlled by advertising and exploited by commercial enterprises.

Caught in this universal conditioning, man too often capitulates and allows himself to be trapped in a net of routines. He loses his natural creativity, though it was lively enough when he was small, even before he started school, an institution which Illich sees as a machine for manufacturing robots for the consumer society. I see it only too clearly in the retired people with whom I am concerned nowadays. Not all of them, I am glad to say. Dr Arthur Jores has pointed out that the crisis of retirement, which is sometimes lethal, is especially threatening to the mind that is deadened by routine, the bureaucratic mind which has renounced all personal life outside the activity of the job itself, now suddenly brought to a full stop.

Though there are so many people who complain about the monotony of their lives, they cling to it more than they realize, because they are so used to it: what would they do if one day the TV were to stop? The State even takes steps to restrict the right of TV personnel to strike. And yet TV has only recently made its appearance. I lived more than half a century without it. What an example of routine – all these people who spend hours every day in front of the little screen, often without giving it much real attention or thought, sometimes dropping off to sleep despite the efforts of the producers to offer worthwhile programmes. Yet they are ready enough to grumble about the programmes, without giving a thought to the fact that if they took an interest in something else it would give them something to do instead of sitting passively there as if they were seeking only to fill up the emptiness of their lives. They could go and play football themselves instead of watching matches from the depths of their armchairs and calling themselves sporting types.

It is clear that routine is ambivalent. We often grumble about it, but we also seek it as an easy alternative to facing up to problems of self-commitment. It is a prison, but also a refuge.

This suggests to me an analogy in which I see an answer to the question raised all through this book. The analogy is a pair of nut-crackers. The shell of the nut represents the protective refuge which has gradually become more hardened as routine has enclosed us in its restricted space. The shell safely encloses the tender tasty fruit of our creative sensibility. Break the nut, and you will discover the fruit inside.

The nut-crackers are all those deprivations (Atlan's noises) which disturb the normal process of life, incarnated, but also fossilized, in routine. The breaking of the nut is a catastrophe as brutal as the unforeseen calamities that strike us. Which of us has not felt himself broken like a little nut by some particularly painful event. Oh! I am a doctor, I am acquainted with men's suffering, and have experienced it myself. I am not trying to reduce it to the cracking of a nut. There is the pain, for which there is no analogy, no scale by which to measure it. I know the importance and the repercussions of the emotional life, always wounded by misfortune, especially by bereavement or by the anguish of seeing a loved one suffering. But it is important to see that there is another aspect of it – a certain disarray caused simply by the need to face a new situation, in which the old routines are no longer going to be of any help. The hard shell is the whole rigid, fixed framework of the genetic code, the psychological complexes, the habits, the prejudices, and the behaviour patterns which imprison us.

Something is broken which will never come together again. And so one begins to ask oneself questions which had tended to get forgotten in the daily round of ordinary life – about the meaning of existence, of suffering, disease, and death. For in our so scientific world no one can explain to us or teach us how to bear adversity. We have to go back to the beginning and feel our way like Jean Piaget's children. Was it not by feeling their way that men slowly searched for God, and is not this what explains the contradictions of the Bible? We find ourselves alone again, alone with ourselves, or with the 'Unknown God' of whom Petru Dumitriu writes, and who remains undefinable. Then it is easier to see how it is that creativity can reappear following trials and deprivations – not that these experiences produce it themselves, but that they make it possible by breaking the old comfortable routines. For creativity is there, hidden, blocked, stifled by all the conventions, but present in our hearts, the gift of God, a constituent of our human nature. The biblical writer expresses this when he says: 'God created man in the image of himself' (Gen. 1.27). God is the Creator. To be in his image is to be endowed with creativity.

Hence the need to create, inborn in every man, his need for adventure. I always remember the remark of one of our boys when he had broken his leg while skiing. He had told us towards the end of the day that he was going to go quickly up to make one last descent. Mechanical ski-lifts (fine routines!) did not yet exist. But since he did not reappear we went to look for him. It was I who found him; and as I bent over him he said in a rather solemn tone of voice, 'At last, something has happened to me!' I was quite surprised. He had felt overprotected, and I had not realized it. He felt that his life was too ordinary to answer his need for creative adventure.

Yes, 'If all were for the best in the best of all possible worlds,' writes Jacques Sarano, 'doubtless man would invent nothing.' And I can quote Atlan once more: 'Noise serves only to permit the realization of the potential constraints contained in the forces of attraction.' The noise of which he is speaking, so small that one might consider it negligible in a rigidly determinist universe, may have immense consequences. He himself quotes Edgar Morin: 'History is nothing but a succession of irremediable disasters.' That is the cracking of the nut. But it can break open of itself. If my nut had fallen to the ground the phenomena of putrefaction would have dealt with the hard shell: the processes of death, which liberate the germ of life and enable it to grow. No new civilization has flourished before its predecessor has crumbled. Now we have the scientists of the Club of Rome announcing disasters, as Jeremiah once did to the Israelites. They are not heeded any more than was he whom André Neher calls 'the Prophet of the Night'.

This, then, is the lesson of our reflections. It is that what disturbs our lives, puts us out, irritates us, annoys us, affects us, makes us suffer – severely sometimes – does not make us grow and develop, but does make growth and development possible, on condition, of course, that we are not destroyed by it, as happens when the nut-crackers are gripped too hard, and the kernel is destroyed along with the shell. Even if the kernel is not destroyed, it always suffers some damage. Before being occasions for creativity, all the ills that man is heir to are grief, pain, and mutilation. That is why we doctors, nurses, social workers, physiotherapists, have a divine vocation to care for them; to study Mother Nature in order to help her in her task, and to understand how she works. For it is nature that heals, as we have known ever since Hippocrates.

I am always astonished by the phenomena of regeneration. When the surgeon inserts his pins and screws and such devices, he is only doing the preparatory work, bringing together the broken pieces of bone. The real work is done by the ordered activity of millions of cells – not a crude stitching together, but invisible mending, fibre by fibre, strand by strand. And when there is a foreign invasion by germs, what a clearing of the decks for action takes place, the whole organism shuddering as the battle commences. It is a very explosion of creativity! A complete communications network is ready, and messages stream out in all directions.

Each cell knows in advance what it must do in the emergency, as if a general could communicate his battle plan to each one of his troops. Each cell has its little code with it, very detailed, one of a print of billions. It knows how to manufacture antibodies. It knows exactly how to distinguish one protein from another, so that in the heat of battle it will not mistake an enemy soldier for an ally. It has learned its code and its alphabet perfectly, for remember it was taught it even before it was born. Much more, it is its very substance, the living matter from which its nucleus is formed, all those nucleic acids, each quite distinct from all the others. There are so few misprints in the code that for a long time scientists believed there were none at all. Now they tell us that when they do happen it is not by chance but to convey even more useful information.

Thus it is that catastrophes and creativity alternate in the lives of nations as in those of individuals, and that every deprivation can be the occasion of a new surge of creativity. We must always let go one thing in order to grasp another. I once used an image for this law of life which many people have remarked upon because they had found it a striking one: it was the image of trapeze artists at the circus, who must let go of their trapeze in time to catch the other. Every catastrophe teaches us something: the doctor never forgets to remind himself of the wrong diagnosis he once made, so as not to make the same mistake again.

Not all deprivations, however, are suffered unwillingly or felt as catastrophes. There are some that are willed, chosen on purpose. A deprivation which a man imposes freely upon himself is a renunciation. Think of the Beatitudes, think of St Francis of Assisi, think of the vow of poverty made by the religious orders. There is a charming remark on the subject of poverty in Elie Wiesel's book *Souls on Fire*. It is so precious, he says, yet 'it costs nothing'. Think of the abandonment of self-will to which every Christian is called. The promise he receives is none other than a new creativity: 'Everyone who has left houses, brothers, sisters, father, mother, children or land for the sake of my name will be repaid a hundred times over' (Matt. 19.29). Jesus often spoke of creativity, with his imagery of trees and fruit, and of vines that are pruned in order to ensure an even more abundant harvest (John 15.2). But the least one can say is that renunciation is no longer in fashion in the West, corrupted as we are by our prosperity.

It is understandable, therefore, that all religions have instituted deprivations in the form of restrictions on sexual activity, such as the prohibition of incest, so dear to Freud, the celibacy of the clergy and, for all, periods of continence or fasts. A religion which demands no renunciation is not taken seriously, and brings no renewal of creativity. Apart from its hygienic value, fasting is a harmless way of bringing about that rupture in the stranglehold of routine of which I was speaking.

I am not so fond of meat that I have to abstain from it. Each of us has his preferences, of which he runs the risk of becoming the prisoner. Thus I have seen pious folk who deprived themselves of all sorts of things, yet could not resist chocolate. My great partiality is for my pipe. Many Christians look upon giving up tobacco as an act of witness to their faith. Following their example I once did so myself. But the time came when I realized that I was being a bit Pharisaical about it, and both my faith and my career put me on guard against that sort of pride. Experience has taught me that the main thing is not what we do or refrain from doing, but the motivation of our acts. A spontaneous decision aimed at expressing my love for God had slipped into the following of a conventional model.

One day much later, I suggested to one of my patients that I would give up smoking along with him, in order to encourage him to do the same. I met him in the street several years later, with a cigarette between his lips.

'So you've taken up smoking again?' I asked.

'I never stopped,' he replied. 'I soon found a doctor who allowed me to smoke.'

'You ought to have told me,' I said to him, 'because I have been off it ever since then.'

But as I parted from him I had a strange feeling of euphoria, which I attributed to the fact that I had been living through a little adventure that had cost nothing, since it had served no purpose.

In the last few years I have come to a better understanding

of the meaning of fasting, and I have decided to abstain from smoking for one month in the year. It costs me hardly any effort, because I do it freely: no one makes me do it. It is only a very small renunciation, but it has a symbolic meaning for me: that of not being the prisoner either of a habit or of a prejudice. Of course I have made renunciations that have been more costly. For instance, when I felt called to change the orientation of my career in order to study the influence on health of the moral and spiritual life. Nobody understood why I was doing this, not even my closest friends. I lost my clientèle, and it was four years before it was replaced. The shell of my professional routine had been broken, but the seed inside was to be slow to germinate.

Who has ever given up a privilege without being forced to do so, except in response to a spiritual call? In his search to discover the motive forces of human behaviour, Freud saw at first only the pleasure principle. Everyone has now recognized the important role which the principle plays in all human actions, from the most selfish to the most generous. But it is impossible to satisfy all one's desires in this world, and Freud himself recognized and described a second principle, that of reality. Reason, it says, bowing to the limitations of reality, imposes renunciation of unattainable desires. What escaped Freud was that there is a third principle, the divine call, which leads to quite other renunciations.

It was not the reality principle which made St Francis of Assisi renounce the privileges of his birth into a rich and powerful family, any more than the Buddha the palace in which he had spent his sheltered childhood, or which led all those monks and nuns, Christians, Jews, Buddhists, Muslims, and other believers, to make a vow of poverty – it was the call of God. And how many of the faithful there are who date their conversion from the moment when they felt themselves broken, like the shell of a nut, in their pride and their obstinacy by the powerful hand of God!

The divine call, however, is a quite personal matter, with the result that there is hardly ever a collective renunciation of some unjust privilege without the pressure of reality in the form of violence. When, on the 4th August 1789, the French nobility renounced its privileges, it was by reason of the popular fury, though it was already too late to assuage it. Neither the freeing of the serfs, nor the emancipation of the slaves, or of women, nor yet the freeing of the colonies, was achieved without bitter confrontations. It is tragic: in the field of history there is no progress possible without the breaking of many shells. However, the courage of exceptional statesmen can play a decisive part, as in the case of Abraham Lincoln in the abolition of slavery, or General De Gaulle in the ending of French domination in Algeria, even though he was put in power by the very people who counted on him to preserve it, and who then looked on him as a traitor.

In all countries parliaments pass law after law, but hardly ever abolish any. Sometimes, indeed, they are to protect the weak, but more often they are aimed at safeguarding the privileges of the powerful. So that the whole system becomes set as a solid block, and any creative initiative comes up against an impenetrable and immovable network of routines. Society becomes like a chequer-board on which it is impossible to play, because every square is already occupied. It was only because the whole country had collapsed that monetary reform became possible in Germany, and the economy was able to take off once more. Each inhabitant started again from scratch with a sum of DM60, and said goodbye to his savings – a sort of vow of poverty imposed on a whole nation. The tragedy of the present North–South dialogue is that the privileged countries are sincerely seeking a solution, but with the proviso that it should not require them to give up anything themselves. It is a utopian aspiration, and one fears that here too it may be too late when we do consent to make some sacrifices.

The conclusion, then, of our reflections, is that in our personal lives as well as in those of nations, there is always suffering, tragedy, deprivation – in short, noise. Such things are always an evil that must be fought against: they have no beneficent virtue in themselves. But precisely because we must combat them, because we must react, and also because in them the mesh of old routines is broken, and our usual models of behaviour no longer serve, we must turn to our innate creativity. That is what can give a new impulse to our lives, one that is more free, more thoughtful, more original, and more fruitful.

Of course there can be no certainty that this will happen, and at the moment of trial it is easy to doubt it. But it is possible, and that very possibility can revive our courage and our hope. That is why I am writing: because if your hope and your courage are restored in this perspective of growth through suffering, the probability of such a favourable outcome is increased, and you have the more reason to fight and to hope. There is a snowball effect.

It is obvious that it is not a matter of certainty, but of probability. You know that modern physics now talks only of probability. It has substituted this more modest concept for the rigorous determinism on which classic physics was based. How much more, then, in the humane sciences must we speak only of probability. It is not certain that your life will become more creative after your present suffering, but it is made the more probable, the more your hope of it has been awakened by so many examples which show that it is possible.

You have noticed that there is always an 'if'. If the orphan has sufficient resources, says Dr Rentchnick; if the deprived person is endowed with a creative mind, says Dr Haynal; if he is given enough help, say I; if noise, says Henri Atlan, instead of causing disorder, and increased entropy, creates and increases order. Yes, the 'ifs' introduce uncertainty, but by the same token they evoke a more or less probable eventuality, and one which becomes the more so, the more it restores your courage. In the end you know that it depends mostly on you and on your own personal attitude.

If anything is certain, it is that every one of life's trials, if only because it breaks the hard crust of our physical and mental habits, creates, like the ploughing of a field, an empty space where seed can be sown. In the sudden void caused by a bereavement, an illness with the contingency of death always possible, failure despite prolonged efforts at success, the return of loneliness when your hope for its banishment has been disappointed, your mind is assailed by fundamental questions to which you hardly ever gave a thought in the coercive whirl of life.

Coercive, and banal: it is frequently the banality of our existence which strikes us when we are brutally brought to a halt in this way. We have protested against the hustle and bustle of modern life. But we have allowed ourselves to be caught in it. Suddenly, so many things that seemed urgent seem so futile. We have sunk into a repetitive routine. We have capitulated in face of the powerful social game which is entirely dedicated to doing rather than being, to success and profit, to know-how and to possession. There is no room left for inspiration in this turmoil, and creativity is inspiration. In order to be truly creative, one must stop to think, to re-think one's personal goal in life, for a man's true work is his life.

I have been impressed to see men thinking such thoughts, even in the midst of success, when some misfortune prompted them. Where might this perpetual climb to power end, even when it is done for the best of causes? They have made me think of the prophet Elijah. He too performed wonders, and in his case it was in God's cause. On Mount Carmel he performed a miracle, aroused the people, and himself slew four hundred and fifty prophets of Baal. But he came up against the powers that were, in the form of Jezebel, who so far from giving way sought to avenge herself and to kill him. Faced with this failure he had to flee and became so depressed that he longed only for death.

Then came the well-known scene. From the depths of a cave in the mountain he heard the majesty of God pass by – at least he heard the successive images of God: first a great hurricane, then an earthquake, then fire. But God himself was not in them, whereas he recognized his presence in 'the sound of a gentle breeze' (I Kings 19.12). Thus, in meditation, the image we have of God is changed. Until then God had seemed to him only the Almighty who crushes his enemies. It was as if he foresaw as Isaiah did, the revelation of Jesus, of God incarnate in a 'servant' . . . 'gentle and humble in heart' (Matt. 11.29), and one who 'does not break the crushed reed' (Isaiah 42.3).

We too, bound up as we are with our technological civilization, have made sacrifice – even in the church – to the quest for power, to the Cartesian illusion of the possibility, using objective reason alone, of arriving at the plenitude of knowledge by the accumulation of things that are sure and certain. We have given priority to the hardness of things over the tenderness of persons. And we have succeeded in constructing a world of things that is extremely highly developed, but to the detriment of the person; an all-powerful mechanical world, in which man himself has become depersonalized. The mechanical, the objective, the repetitive, that is the world of things. It is the person which is endowed with creativity, with fantasy, poetry, and feeling. We have put our faith in technological progress, in the progress of things.

The Christian hope which inspires me is not a thing, but a person – not that little thing 'the poor consolation dispensed to humankind', as the Greeks thought, forgotten at the bottom of Pandora's box, and so escaping the dispersal of the contents when her curiosity prompted her to open it; nor the grand discovery on the threshold of which Renan believed science to be standing, which would put an end to all uncertainty about the mystery of the universe – no, a person. The person of Jesus, who though he was the Son of the Father, had to feel his way to know the Father's will, but who is alive, whereas we are all going towards death, and who is awaiting us beyond death, where he told us that he would prepare a place for us (John 14.2).

List of Works Quoted

Assagioli, Roberto, *Psychosynthesis*, Turnstone Press 1975.
Atlan, Henri, *Entre le cristal et la fumée: essai sur l'organisation du vivant*, Le Seuil, Paris 1979.
—*L'organisation biologique et la théorie de l'information*, Hermann, Paris 1972.
Augustine, Saint, *The Confessions*, Nelson 1938.
Babel, Henry, *Le secret des grandes religions*, La Baconnière, Neuchâtel 1975.
Balint, Michael, *The Doctor, his Patient and the Illness*, Pitman Books 1968.
Benoît, Jean-Daniel, *Calvin, directeur d'âmes*, Oberlin, Strasbourg.
Bovet, Théodore, *Le mariage, ce grand mystère*, Delachaux & Niestlé, Neuchâtel 1956.
Chabanis, Christian, *Dieu existe? – Oui*, Stock, Paris 1979.
Charon, Jean E., *L'esprit, cet inconnu*, Collection Marabout, Albin Michel, Paris 1977.
Chouraqui, André, *La Bible*, trs into French, complete in 26 Vols., Desclée de Brouwer, Paris 1974–77.
—*Ce que je crois*, Grasset, Paris 1979.
Collins, Gary R., *The Christian Psychology of Paul Tournier*, Baker Book house, Grand Rapids, Michigan 1973.
Dawkins, Richard, *The Selfish Gene*, OUP 1976.
Delaunay, Albert, see Chabanis, C.
Delumeau, Jean, *La peur en Occident*, Fayard, Paris 1978.
Descartes, René, *Discourse on Method and Other Writings*, trs F. E. Sutcliffe, Penguin Classics 1970.
Dolto, Françoise, *Dominique, Analysis of an Adolescent*, trs I. Kats, Souvenir Press 1974.
Dröscher, Vitus B., *They Love and Kill*, trs J. V. Heurck, Dutton, New York 1976, and W. H. Allen, London 1977.
Dubois, Paul, *Les psychonévroses et leur traitement moral*, Masson, Paris 1905.
Dumitriu, Petru, *Au Dieu inconnu*, Le Seuil, Paris 1979.

Creative Suffering

Duruz, Didier, *Une errance au pays du vieillir . . . approche existentielle et réflexion*, a research study, *Institut d'Etudes Socialies*, Geneva, 21 Oct. 1980.
Fabre, Jean-Henri, *Insect Life: Souvenirs of a Naturalist*, ed. F. Merrifield, Macmillan 1901.
Foerster, H. von, *On Self-Organising Systems and their Environments*, Yovitz & Cameron, Pergamon Press 1960.
Foucault, Michel, *The Order of Things*, Tavistock Publications 1970.
Fouché, Suzanne, *Souffrance, école de vie*, Spes, Paris 1959.
Frankl, Viktor E., *La psychothérapie et son image de l'homme*, Resma, Paris 1970.
Freud, Sigmund, 'Mourning and Melancholy', *The Standard Edition of the Complete Psychological Works of Sigmund Freud*, Vol. 14, Hogarth Press 1953.
—*Beyond the Pleasure Principle*, Hogarth Press and Institute of Psychoanalysis, London 1950.
—*Totem and Taboo*, trs J. Strachey, Routledge 1950.
—*The Future of an Illusion*, ed. J. Strachey, trs W. D. R. Scott, International Psychoanalytical Library, Hogarth Press 1962.
—*Moses and Monotheism*, trs K. Jones, Hogarth Press 1951.
Fromm, Erich, 'The Creative Attitude', quoted in M. Philibert, *L'échelle des âges*, Le Seuil, Paris 1968.
—*The Art of Loving*, Allen & Unwin 1957.
Fuchs, Eric, *Le désir et la tendresse*, Labor et Fides, Geneva 1979.
Gander, Joseph, 'Die Entwicklung der Medizin von Virchow zu Tournier', *Civitas*, Year I No. 9.
Girard, René, *Deceit, Desire, and the Novel*, trs Y. Freccero, Johns Hopkins Press, Baltimore and London 1969.
Glucksmann, André, *Master Thinkers*, Harvester Press 1980.
Gonseth, Ferdinand, *Déterminisme et libre-arbitre*, Editions du Griffon, Neuchâtel 1944.
Goudot-Perret, Andrée, 'Cybernétique et biologie', *Que sais-je?* No. 1257, Presses Universitaires de France, Paris 1973.
Granjon, Pierre, *Qu'est-ce que la guérison?*, Berger-Levrault, Paris 1956.
Grimal, Pierre, 'La mythologie grecque', *Que sais-je?* No. 582, Presses Universitaires de France, Paris 1953.
Guernier, Maurice, *Tiers monde: trois quarts du monde*, Report to the Club of Rome, Dunod-Bordas, Paris 1980.

List of Works Quoted

Gusdorf, Georges, *Dialogue avec le médecin*, Labor et Fides, Geneva 1962.

Haynal, André, 'Discours psychanalytique sur le manque', in Rentchnick, *Les orphelins mènent-ils le monde?* (q.v.).

Horn, Frances, *Psychothérapie des cancéreux*, a paper read at the Conference on the Medicine of the Person, Bad Boll 1976.

Huebschmann, Heinrich, 'Ueber die Zweideutigkeit des Wohlbefindes bei organisch Kranken am Beispiel von zwei Patienten mit Hertzinfakt', *Gesundheitspolitik*, Berlin 1961 Pt. 4.

Illich, Ivan, *Medical Nemesis*, Calder & Boyars 1975.

—*Tools for Conviviality*, Calder & Boyars 1973.

Janov, Arthur, *The Primal Scream*, Abacus Books, Sphere Books 1973.

Jaspers, Karl, *Great Philosophers*, trs R. Manheim, Harcourt Brace 1975.

Jores, Arthur, and Puchta, H. G., *Der Pensionieurungstod*, München-Berlin Medizinische Klinik 1959.

Jung, C. G., *Collected Works*, Routledge & Kegan Paul 1953.

Kaiser, Edmond, *La marche aux enfants*, Editions Pierre-Marcel Favre, Lausanne 1979.

Klein, Melanie, *Envy and Gratitude and other works 1946–63*, Vol. 4, Dell Publishing Co., New York 1977.

Klopfenstein, Freddy, *Le soleil est nouveau tous les jours*, La Baconnière, Neuchâtel 1977.

Kubler-Ross, Elisabeth, *Living with Death and Dying*, Souvenir Press 1981.

Kurimura, Michio, *La communion des Saints dans l'oeuvre de Paul Claudel*, Ed. France Tosho, Tokyo.

Lagache, 'Le travail de deuil', *Revue Française de Psychanalyse*, X, 4, 1938.

Lechler, Walter, and Lair, Jacqueline Cary, *I Exist, I Need, I am Entitled: A Story of Love, Courage, and Survival*, Doubleday, Garden City, NY 1980.

Maeder, Alphonse, *La personne du médecin, un agent psychothérapeutique*, Delachaux & Niestlé, Neuchâtel 1953.

Martin, Bernard, *The Healing Ministry in the Church*, trs M. Clement, Lutterworth Press 1960.

—'Si le médecin se laisse mettre en question', *La vie protestante*, Geneva, 14 Jan. 1977.

Maurois, André, 'Otages du destin', *Cahiers Ladapt*, Paris, No. 65, 15 Feb. 1979.

Milton, John, *Paradise Lost*, CUP 1972–76.

Missenard, André, *A la recherche du temps et du rythme*, Plon, Paris 1940.

Monod, Jacques, *Chance and Necessity*, trs A. Wainhouse, Fontana 1974.

Morel, Bernard, *Cybernétique et transcendance*, Vieux Colombier, Paris 1964.

Morin, Edgar, *Le paradigne perdu: la nature humaine*, Le Seuil, Paris 1973.

Mottu, Philippe, *Le serpent dans l'ordinateur*, La Baconnière, Neuchâtel 1974.

Mounier, Emmanuel, 'Médecine, quatrième pouvoir?', *Esprit*, March 1950.

Nef, Frida, *Un sens à la vie*, Editions de Caux, CH 1978.

Neher, André, *Jérémie*, Plon, Paris 1960.

Odier, Charles, *Les deux sources, consciente et inconsciente, de la vie morale*, La Baconnière, Neuchâtel 1943.

Peaston, Monroe, *Personal Living: An Introduction to Paul Tournier*, Harper & Row, New York 1972.

Piaget, Jean, *The Origin of Intelligence in the Child*, trs M. Cook, Routledge & Kegan Paul 1953.

Plattner, Paul, *Glücklichere Ehen*, Huber, Berne 1950.

Porret, Jean-Marie, *Orphelinage et créativité*, Doctoral Thesis in the University of Geneva, 1977.

Racanelli, Francesco, *La souffrance vaincue*, Delachaux & Niestlé, Neuchâtel 1954.

Renard, Jules, *Carrots*, trs from the French (*Poil-de-Carotte*) by G. W. Stonier, Grey Walls Press 1946.

Rentchnick, Pierre, and Accoce, Pierre, *Ces malades qui nous gouvernent*, Stock, Paris 1976.

—*Les orphelins mènent-ils le monde?*, with additional essays by De Senarclens, Pierre, and Haynal, André, Stock, Paris 1978.

—'Les orphelins mènent le monde', *Médecine et Hygiène*, Geneva, No. 1171, 26 Nov. 1975.

Richardeau, M., *Bible et psychanalyse 3: le personnage de Moïse*, a cassette issued by Union des Groupes Bibliques Universitaires de France, 21 Rue Serpente, Paris.

List of Works Quoted

Ricoeur, Paul, *History and Truth*, trs C. A. Kelbley, Northwestern UP, Evanston 1965.

—' "Morale sans péché" ou péché sans moralisme', *Esprit* Aug.-Sept. 1954.

—*Freud and Philosophy. An Essay on Interpretation*, trs D. Savage, Yale University Press, New Haven & London 1970.

Riesman, David, *The Solitary Crowd*, Yale UP, New Haven 1961.

Rogers, Carl R., *On Becoming a Person*, Constable 1961.

Rousseau, Jean-Jacques, *Lettre à Malesherbes*.

Sadat, Anwar, *In Search of Identity: an Autobiography*, Harper & Row, New York 1979.

Sarano, Jacques, *L'homme double – dualité et duplicité*, L'Epi, Paris 1979.

—'Sur Illich. Nemesis médicale', *Esprit* 1977, No. 2.

Sartre, Jean-Paul, *Words*, trs Irene Clephane, Penguin Books in association with Hamish Hamilton 1967.

Senarclens, Pierre de, 'La biographie psychanalytique des hommes politiques est-elle réalisable?', in Rentchnick, *Les orphelins mènent-ils le monde?* (q.v.).

Shannon, C. E., and Weaver, *The Mathematical Theory of Communication*, University of Illinois Press, Urbana, Ill. 1949.

Solzhenitsyn, Alexander, 'A World Split Apart', *Solzhenitsyn at Harvard*, ed. Ronald Berman, Ethics and Public Policy Center, Washington, DC 1980.

Sorokine, Pitirim, *The American Sex Revolution*, Porter Sargent, Boston.

Sosnowski, Richard, *Retraite, esseulement: il y a solitude et solitude*, Unpublished Bible-study at the Conference on the Medicine of the Person, Warwick 1980.

Starobinski, Jean, *Jean-Jacques Rousseau, la transparence et l'obstacle*, Plon, Paris 1957.

Tournier, Paul, *The Violence Inside*, trs Edwin Hudson, SCM Press 1978.

—*Mutig leben*, Reinhardt, Basel 1980.

—*The Gift of Feeling*, trs Edwin Hudson, SCM Press 1981.

—*To Resist or to Surrender?*, trs G. S. Gilmour, SCM Press 1965.

—*The Meaning of Persons*, trs Edwin Hudson, SCM Press 1957.

—*The Healing of Persons*, trs Edwin Hudson, Harper & Row, New York 1965.

Unwin, J. D., *Sex and Culture*, OUP 1934.
Verges, A., 'Faute et liberté', *Annales universitaires*, Besançon, Vol. 10, 1969.
Wiesel, Elie, *Souls on Fire: Portraits and Legends of Hassidic Masters*, trs M. Wiesel, Weidenfeld & Nicolson 1972.
Ziegler, Jean, *Les vivants et la mort*, Le Seuil, Paris 1975.
Zorn, Fritz, *Mars*, trs Robert and Rita Kimber, Alfred A. Knopf, New York 1982.